T0220339

THE MEDICAL EXAMINER SERVICE

THE MEDICAL EXAMINER SERVICE

A Practical Guide for England and Wales

Jason Payne-James
LLM MSc FFFLM FRCS FRCP FCSFS
FFCFM(RCPA) RCPathME DFM
LBIPP Mediator
Specialist in Forensic & Legal Medicine
& Consultant Forensic Physician
Lead Medical Examiner
Norfolk & Norwich University Hospital
Honorary Clinical Professor
William Harvey Research Institute
Queen Mary University of London
London, UK

Suzy Lishman CBE FRCPath RCPathME
Consultant Histopathologist
and Lead Medical Examiner
North-West Anglia NHS Foundation Trust
Chair
Medical Examiners Committee
The Royal College of Pathologists
London, UK

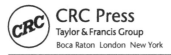

CRC Press
Taylor & Francis Group
Boca Raton London New York

CRC Press is an imprint of the
Taylor & Francis Group, an **informa** business

First edition published 2023
by CRC Press
6000 Broken Sound Parkway NW, Suite 300, Boca Raton, FL 33487-2742

and by CRC Press
4 Park Square, Milton Park, Abingdon, Oxon, OX14 4RN

CRC Press is an imprint of Taylor & Francis Group, LLC

Library of Congress Cataloging-in-Publication Data
Names: Payne-James, Jason, editor. | Lishman, Suzy, editor.
Title: The medical examiner service : a practical guide for England and Wales / edited by Jason Payne-James, Suzannah Lishman.
Description: First edition. | Boca Raton : CRC Press, 2022. | Includes bibliographical references and index. | Summary: "This book provides a practical guide for all those working in or with Medical Examiner Services in England and Wales. It is an adjunct to the e-learning and face-to-face training required to fulfil the Medical Examiner and Medical Examiner Officer roles. Medical Examiner Services also work closely with a wide range of stakeholders including bereavement and mortuary teams, Coroners and their Officers, Registrars, Funeral Directors and those working in clinical governance and patient safety. This book provides an essential overview of all aspects of the Medical Examiner system for anyone working in these areas, or in any aspect of the support and management of the deceased and bereaved. A concise guide including the knowledge base required to develop and run a Medical Examiner Service Content is completely aligned with required training Written by those with direct experience of establishing and working with Medical Examiner Services Relevant to a wide range of stakeholders who work with patients and the bereaved"— Provided by publisher.
Identifiers: LCCN 2021050513 | ISBN 9781032004198 (paperback) | ISBN 9781032037394 (hardback) | ISBN 9781003188759 (ebook)
Subjects: MESH: Coroners and Medical Examiners | Cause of Death | State Medicine | Social Support | England | Wales
Classification: LCC RA1063.4 | NLM W 800 | DDC 614/.1—dc23/eng/20211101
LC record available at https://lccn.loc.gov/2021050513

ISBN: 978-1-032-03739-4 (hbk)
ISBN: 978-1-032-00419-8 (pbk)
ISBN: 978-1-003-18875-9 (ebk)

DOI: 10.1201/9781003188759

Typeset in Times New Roman
by Apex CoVantage, LLC

Contents

Foreword

The publication of *The Medical Examiner Service – A Practical Guide for England and Wales* is a significant milestone in the establishment of the Medical Examiner service. As editors and authors, Jason Payne-James and Suzy Lishman have brought together considerable knowledge and experience in one place. In any new medical service, 'The Book' is a marker that the service has arrived and is here to stay.

At the time of publication, the Medical Examiner service is not yet fully implemented; it is in a non-statutory phase, with the full design of the statutory service to be settled by Parliament. Therefore, this book must be regarded as a work-in-progress but a valuable reference resource to Medical Examiners and Medical Examiner Officers nonetheless. It is complementary to my *Good Practice Guidelines*, published in January 2020.

Nearly two decades have passed since Medical Examiners were first recommended by Dame Janet Smith in her *The Shipman Inquiry Third Report: Death Certification and the Investigation of Deaths by Coroners* but the reasons for implementation are as relevant as ever, especially to the families of those bereaved as a result of the murders committed by Harold Shipman.

Pilot sites for the Medical Examiner service showed benefits for bereaved people, giving them a voice at a time of critical importance in their lives, as well as providing consistency and accuracy of cause of death and coroner notification. These benefits are now consistently realised throughout England and Wales after implementation began in 2019.

Since 2008, pioneers of the Medical Examiner service, as pilots or early adopters in Sheffield, Gloucestershire, mid-Essex, Powys, Brighton and Hove, Birmingham, inner north London, and Leicester doggedly maintained the case for a Medical Examiner service. They held bereaved people at the centre of the process as I do now, and it is essential this connection is never diluted. This is reflected in the chapters of this book.

The *Medical Examiner Service – A Practical Guide for England and Wales* correctly emphasises the importance of Medical Examiner Officers, who are the primary contact for stakeholders. Establishing links to stakeholders is key to the Medical Examiner service. This book will be relevant to a wide range of professionals including doctors certifying deaths, palliative care teams, Coroners, Coroner's officers, Registrars of births and deaths and those working in the funeral industry.

Building on the remarkable success of the implementation of the non-statutory Medical Examiner service, it is my expectation that the transition to the statutory service will be as smooth as possible maintaining the principles and practices set out in this book. Success is thanks to very many committed colleagues, including the authors and editors of this book. This is their opportunity to consolidate work to date and to shape the future.

Few have the opportunity to create a new medical specialty, a nationally comprehensive service improvement, or touch the lives of bereaved people in a positive way. It is a great privilege to lead this service.

Jason Payne-James and Suzy Lishman have a wealth of editorial and Medical Examiner experience. They have done a splendid job with this first-ever textbook of the Medical Examiner service in England and Wales.

The Medical Examiner service in England and Wales is becoming a critical part of the most comprehensive and careful mortality review service in the world. The benefits will show in time, but bereaved people will remain front and centre as principal beneficiaries.

Dr Alan Fletcher
National Medical Examiner

Preface

This book gives an outline of the new Medical Examiner service in England & Wales, and its relationship to, and information about, those other services and professions that are intimately involved in the care, management and support of the deceased and bereaved.

The rationale for the Medical Examiner service is to ensure that the concerns of the bereaved and others involved in the care of the deceased are identified and acted upon, whilst simultaneously improving the quality of Medical Certificates of Cause of Death. Although long in gestation, the growth and development of a Medical Examiner Services in acute hospitals and health boards across England & Wales has, since May 2019, been rapid and dramatic, and, if anything, has been unexpectedly enhanced by the COVID-19 pandemic, which started within one year of its introduction.

The Medical Examiner service can be considered to be in its adolescence, but growing and expanding with speed, towards the ultimate goal of reviewing every non-coronial death in England and Wales, wherever it takes place. The integration of a completely new element of the medicolegal review of death has been made possible by the enthusiasm of Medical Examiners and Medical Examiner Officers within the service, but equally by the support and patience of the myriad of individuals and teams who have daily contact with the deceased and bereaved. Much of the compassion, knowledge and skills of those individuals and teams is often unseen and unrecognised. We hope this book will go some way to ensuring that this is no longer the case.

This book provides information from those who have been involved in the development and training of Medical Examiners and Medical Examiner Officers, but additionally, and most importantly, from those with direct experience of the services about which they write, and their personal and varied experiences.

The book is not a rigid 'how to' guide, but one that uses examples of the needs of each area considered to identify how things can be done. There is substantial variation in how Medical Examiner Services have, and are developing, and this may be dependent on a huge variety of local factors, impacting on and impacted by different approaches. It is best to assume that there is rarely one single correct way to deal with most challenges, and that the key to developing a workable consensus is by discussion and communication with other services.

The Chief Coroner has stated '*Medical Examiners are now part of the wider death oversight and investigation system in England and Wales. Their duties are different to coroners but they are the counterpart for coroners and coroners and their staff should work in a spirit of partnership and mutual respect with the Medical Examiners*'. We believe that the development of the Medical Examiner service could be one of the most significant developments impacting on patient care and safety but, most importantly, will ensure that the voices of the deceased and bereaved are clearly heard.

Jason Payne-James, Southminster
Suzy Lishman, Rutland

Acknowledgements

The editors wish to thank Nora Naughton, Sam Thompson and Grace Payne-James for their invaluable support and hard work in the development and production of this book.

Contributors

Gabriel Callaghan
MPhys(Hons) MSc
Auditor and Analyst

Nigel Callaghan LLB (Hons) LMSSA (Lond)
T (GP) FP Cert DipPnMed FFFLM MFSSoc
MCI Arb RCPathME
Consultant Forensic Physician and
    Barrister
Faculty of Forensic and Legal Medicine
Judiciary
Durham, UK

Katie A Carpenter MBBS MRCGP
FRCP LLM RCPath ME
Medical Examiner
Norfolk and Norwich University Hospitals
    NHS Foundation Trust
Norfolk, UK

Siobhan Costello
Regional Medical Examiner Officer
NHS England / Improvement East of
    England Region
Cambridge, UK

Daniel Elton
Government, Regional and Religious
    Affairs Officer
Board of Deputies of British Jews
London, UK

C George M Fernie LLB MBChB MPhil
FFFLM FRCGP FRFCPE
FRCP DFM
Senior Medical Reviewer
Healthcare Improvement Scotland
Edinburgh, UK

Meryl Hepple
Manager
Bereavement Office

Norfolk and Norwich University Hospitals
NHS Foundation Trust
Norwich, UK

Nigel L Kennea MBBChir PhD
FRCPCH RCPath (ME)
Consultant Neonatologist and Lead
Medical Examiner
St George's University Hospitals NHS
    Foundation Trust
London, UK

Suzy Lishman CBE FRCPath RCPathME
Consultant Histopathologist and
    Lead Medical Examiner
North-West Anglia NHS Foundation Trust
and
Chair
Medical Examiners Committee
The Royal College of Pathologists
London, UK

Berenice Lopez MRCP FRCGP FRCPath
Associate Medical Director Quality and
    Safety
Consultant Chemical Pathologist
    (Metabolic Medicine)
Norfolk and Norwich University Hospitals
    NHS Foundation Trust
Norwich
and
RCPath Clinical Director Quality and
    Safety
Royal College of Pathologists
London, UK

Ellen Makings
MBBS FRCA FFICM RCPathME
Regional Medical Examiner
    Medical Director System
    Improvement
NHS England / Improvement East of
    England Region and Lead Medical
    Examiner Royal Papworth Hospital
Cambridge, UK

Paul Marks BA LLM MD FRCS PFFLM RCPathME
Professor
HM Senior Coroner for the City of
  Kingston Upon Hull & the County of the
  East Riding of Yorkshire
Hull Coroner's Court & Office
Hull, UK

Mohamed Omer MBE
Board Member
Gardens of Peace Muslim Cemetery
Chair, National Burial Council
Ilford, UK

Louise Parapanos BA BSc (Hons)
Lead Medical Examiner Officer
Norfolk and Norwich University Hospital
Norwich, UK

Brian Parsons BA PhD Dip FD MBIE AICCM
Funeral Director, Researcher and Funeral
  Historian
Funeral Service Training [London]
London UK

Jason Payne-James
LLM MSc FFFLM FRCS FRCP FCSFS FFCFM(RCPA) RCPathME DFM LBIPP Mediator
Specialist in Forensic & Legal Medicine
  & Consultant Forensic Physician
Lead Medical Examiner
Norfolk & Norwich University Hospital
and
Honorary Clinical Professor
William Harvey Research Institute
Queen Mary University of London
London, UK

John Pitchers MSc FAAPT FRSPH MIBMS
Service Manager
Mortuary and Coroner Support
HTA Designated Individual
  and Chair
Association of Anatomical Pathology
  Technology
Bristol, UK

Daisy Shale MSc Csci FIBMS RCPathMEO
Lead Medical Examiner Officer for Wales
Office of the Lead Medical Examiner for
  Wales
St Asaph, Wales

Jason Shannon BSc MB ChB FRCPath RCPathME
Consultant Pathologist
Cwm Taf Morgannwg University Health
  Board
and Lead Medical Examiner for Wales
NHS Wales Shared Services Partnership
Mamhilad, Wales

Golda Shelley-Fraser MBChB FRCPath RCPathME
Regional Medical Examiner
South West of England
NHS England and Improvement
and
Consultant Histopathologist
Royal United Hospital Bath NHS
  Foundation Trust
Bath, UK

Deborah Smith
Registrar of Births, Deaths, Marriages and
  Civil Partnerships
King's Lynn Town Hall
King's Lynn, UK

CHAPTER 1

Background to the Medical Examiner Service in England and Wales

Jason Payne-James and Suzy Lishman

Introduction

It is important, although may appear strange, to have to explain in the introductory paragraph of a book on the Medical Examiner system what the term means, but 'medical examiner' has a different meaning in different jurisdictions. This book explores the Medical Examiner system in England and Wales, which was introduced in 2019 to scrutinise all non-coronial deaths. Medical Examiners in England and Wales are registered medical practitioners from a wide variety of clinical backgrounds. In some jurisdictions, the term solely refers to forensic pathologists undertaking post mortem examinations.

Similarly, an explanation is needed to ensure that the role of Her Majesty's Coroner (HM Coroner) in England and Wales is not confused with other coronial systems in other jurisdictions. In England and Wales, a Coroner holds a judicial post and requires legal experience and qualifications. The office of Coroner was originally established in 1194 as a form of tax collector but, over the centuries, has evolved into an independent judicial officer, responsible for the investigation of sudden, violent or unnatural death.

The Medical Examiner (ME) system was introduced in England and Wales in April 2019 after a decade or so of pilot studies. In this system, an ME in England and Wales is an independent, senior doctor who scrutinises (reviews) deaths that are not investigated by the England and Wales coronial system. Thus, the ME system in England and Wales is now an essential part of the medicolegal investigation for deaths that are not overseen by the coronial system (the majority of deaths). The ME system works very closely with coronial services. There were more than 500 000 deaths in England and Wales in 2019[1] and more than 200 000 of these were notified to Her Majesty's (HM) Coroners, of which over 80 000 had post-mortem examinations.[2] Those not reported to HM Coroners will all, in future, be reviewed by the Medical Examiner system. Overall numbers of deaths for 2020/2021 have been distorted upwards by the coronavirus pandemic and are in excess of 600 000. In England, the ME system was initially introduced in acute hospitals scrutinising hospital deaths, and is now being extended to cover all non-coronial deaths by 2023. In Wales, deaths in the community have been reviewed since the outset.

DOI: 10.1201/9781003188759-1

1

This chapter explains the role, function and aims of the Medical Examiner system in England and Wales. This system has been established to improve and fill gaps in the medicolegal investigation of death. It has been developed to address perceived gaps in review of all deaths, to identify patient safety issues, and to prevent previously identified scenarios where the concerns of families and whistleblowers about care of the deceased have been ignored. The Medical Examiner system is currently on a non-statutory footing but that is likely to change to a statutory basis by April 2023, recognising the need for all relevant government departments to be ready and aligned to enable successful implementation. This will be centrally funded in England following the required amendment to the Coroners and Justice Act 2009, via the Health and Care Act 2022, confirming Medical Examiners in England will be hosted in NHS bodies rather than local authorities.[3]

Concerns about the Medicolegal Investigation of Death

There have been many concerns expressed over the years about the medicolegal investigation of death, and a large number of UK reports and committees have identified shortcomings in the process. In particular, such reports have indicated that opportunities for improving patient safety have been missed and the potential for concealed homicide is present.

An Inquiry by the UK House of Commons Constitutional Affairs Committee stated: *'This Inquiry was set up to investigate the systems of death certification and investigation in England and Wales against a background of continued inaction by the Government in response to two reports published in 2003: Death Certification and the Investigation of Deaths by Coroners, the 3rd Report of the Shipman Inquiry under Dame Janet Smith (the "Shipman Inquiry"); and Death Certification and Investigation in England, Wales and Northern Ireland: The Report of a Fundamental Review 2003 under Tom Luce (the "Luce Review"). Both reports found the systems for the certification and investigation of deaths in England and Wales to be unfit for modern society'.*[4]

All doctors in the United Kingdom should be aware of Harold Shipman, an apparently respected general practitioner from Hyde in Greater Manchester, UK, who, over a period of 20 or more years, was responsible for the murder of around 250 of his patients. On 31 January 2000, he was found guilty of murdering 15 patients and was sentenced to life imprisonment. He died by suicide in prison on 13 January 2004. The murders raised two main questions – what was his motive and, most significantly, why did nobody in authority realise what was happening?[5] The Shipman Inquiry was initiated to investigate his activities and it established that he was able to conceal malpractice and kill many of his patients because the systems in place permitted him to avoid questions being asked as he was able to certify the causes of death of so many patients without scrutiny.

The Shipman Inquiry was set up in January 2001. The Inquiry had a broad remit and was tasked with investigating the extent of Shipman's unlawful activities, enquiring into the activities of the statutory authorities and other organisations involved, and making recommendations on the steps needed to protect patients in the future. In a series of reports published between 2001 and 2003, the Inquiry made a number of recommendations for the reform of various British systems. It called for Coroners to be better trained and underlined that better controls on the use of Schedule 2, 3 and 4 drugs by doctors and pharmacists were needed. It also recommended that fundamental changes be implemented in the way that doctors are overseen by the General Medical Council.

The Inquiry also established that there were flaws in the system for reviewing cremations where doctors ('medical referees'), whose role was to independently review the cause of death,[6] did not recognise Dr Shipman as anything but a respected colleague and thus enabled acceptance of his dishonest accounts of his patients' deaths without question. For those patients undergoing burials, Dr Shipman was not required to consult any other medical practitioner and the lack of medical knowledge of registrars of births and deaths meant that the causes of death he proposed were accepted and registered without question. The system, as it was, depended on the integrity and honesty of the doctor and there was no robust and independent oversight. These concerns reiterated and reinforced those of other reports and inquiries, which had also noted that existing arrangements for death certification were confusing and provided inadequate safeguards against possible criminal activity.

The term 'Medical Examiner' is referred to at para 17.29 of Dame Janet Smith's third report,[7] in which reference is made to establishing the role of Medical Coroner ('*17.29 The Society of Registration Officers suggested that the office of medical Coroner should be a statutory post, independent from the NHS, with accountability passing up to a Chief Medical Coroner (the Society favoured the term "Medical Examiner")* at the head of a free-standing national agency'. That same report also referred to the Finnish system of death certification in the following terms: '*18.122 The most impressive aspect of the Finnish system of death certification was the emphasis on the importance of accurately ascertaining the cause of death, even where the death was apparently natural. This is of considerable significance, not only for the deceased's family, but also for society generally; it has significant implications for public health*'.

The Shipman Inquiry recommended that a new national Coroners' service under a Chief Coroner should be established at arm's length from national government, replacing the system of local Coroners appointed and funded by local authorities. This service would be responsible for the final certification of death and for deciding whether further investigation was necessary in all deaths. The new system would include both medical Coroners, who would be responsible for

Table 1.1   Relevant sections in the 2009 Coroners and Justice Act introducing the Medical Examiner into legislation

19	Medical Examiners
(1)	[Local authorities] (in England) and Local Health Boards (in Wales) must appoint persons as Medical Examiners to discharge the functions conferred on Medical Examiners by or under this Chapter.
(2)	Each [local authority] or Board must—
	(a) appoint enough Medical Examiners, and make available enough funds and other resources, to enable those functions to be discharged in its area;
	(b) monitor the performance of Medical Examiners appointed by the [local authority] or Board by reference to any standards or levels of performance that those examiners are expected to attain.
(3)	A person may be appointed as a Medical Examiner only if, at the time of the appointment, he or she—
	(c) is a registered medical practitioner and has been throughout the previous 5 years, and
	(b) practises as such or has done within the previous 5 years.

establishing the medical cause of death, and judicial Coroners, who would carry out further investigations where necessary (e.g. in the case of suspicious deaths). It was this proposed role of 'Medical Coroner' that evolved into the present Medical Examiner, with the role of Medical Examiner formally introduced to the England and Wales jurisdiction by the Coroners and Justice Act 2009 (Table 1.1).[8] The Department of Health had proposed in a consultation: *'The Third Report of the Shipman Inquiry Chaired by Dame Janet Smith drew attention to the difference in the arrangements for death certification between cremations and burials. While a series of checks is made before a body can be released for cremation, a single certificate is required for burial. The Government considers that these different arrangements are no longer justified and is proposing to introduce a single system for death certification for both cremations and burials. The proposed arrangements are intended to provide a common level of assurance to all bereaved families that there were no suspicious circumstances surrounding the death, while simplifying the administrative process. They will also improve public health surveillance of cause of death. The new arrangements will be overseen by a Medical Examiner attached to a local Primary Care Trust (or an equivalent organisation in Wales).'*[9]

The 'Luce Review' (Death Certification and Investigation in England, Wales and Northern Ireland: The report of a fundamental review 2003[10]) came to broadly similar conclusions to the Shipman Inquiry. However, it was to be more than 20 years after Harold Shipman was convicted and 10 years after the Coroners and Justice Act before a national rollout of Medical Examiners was begun, and then not in the structure initially envisaged.[11,12] As long ago as 2007, Tom Luce commented: *'In many respects the government's reform package has sensible aims, which doctors and all informed opinion would support – modernising the ancient and long neglected Coroner system, abolishing single doctor certification in burial cases and the elaborate extra process for cremations, introducing monitoring and support for the death certification process, and improving links between death regulation and public health analysis. . . . With much important detail still to settle, legislation to enact, and implementation to deliver, no one can accuse the government of excessive haste.'*[8]

Detail was still being considered, as shown in a letter from the Department of Health Lead Regional Director for Death Certification Reforms (2012)[13] who advised that there were still important, unresolved issues, namely:

- *'The collection of the Medical Examiner fee continues to be a challenge. The costs associated with collecting the fee have a direct bearing on the fee that the public may need to pay if the funding option for the Medical Examiner service continues to be funds generated by the Medical Examiner fee. . . . All the options have raised issues for further consideration.*
- *'On the non-forensic external examination of the body, the Death Certification Steering Group recently endorsed a proposal that someone with suitable expertise other than a medical practitioner can undertake the examination and provide assurances for families that anything untoward will come to light, including neglect and poor standards of care. I should add that certifying doctors completing a MCCD will continue to have the option to examine a body.*
- *'The third issue is about developing appropriate Medical Examiner's service standards and Medical Examiner's performance standards and procedures. We want to avoid unnecessary burden on local authorities and as such, the service standards must be appropriate and have measurable indicators. Similarly, standards and procedures for Medical Examiners should enable peer-review and self-audit by Medical Examiners. Worth noting, is that local authorities will have no role in assessing Medical Examiners in their professional capacity, in fact primary legislation prohibits it. The consultation document will explore broad headings for both sets of standards.'*

In the interim, other hospital-based scandals were the subject of major inquiries.

Hospital Inquiries and Drivers for Implementation

Perhaps the most significant driver for the (at that time non-existent) Medical Examiner system was the 2013 Report of the Mid Staffordshire NHS Foundation Trust Public Inquiry,[14] chaired by (now Sir) Robert Francis QC, which identified numerous, serious failings in care between 2005 and 2009. The report made 290 recommendations, of which a number made specific reference to the need for an independent Medical Examiner system. Table 1.2 shows its recommendations regarding Medical Examiners. The report recognised that *'Significant changes have occurred in the coronial court system since the events under review, including the appointment of a Chief Coroner and the creation of the new post of Independent Medical Examiner (IME)'.*

Other hospital-based scandals have highlighted poor care or deaths that may have been prevented had an effective system of independent scrutiny been in place.

The Report of the Morecambe Bay Investigation in 2015, which was to examine concerns raised by the occurrence of serious incidents in maternity services,

Table 1.2 Recommendations from the 2013 Report of the Mid Staffordshire NHS Foundation Trust Public Inquiry relating to Medical Examiners

Number	Theme	Recommendation
275	Independent Medical Examiners	It is of considerable importance that independent Medical Examiners are independent of the organisation whose patients' deaths are being scrutinised.
276		Sufficient numbers of independent Medical Examiners need to be appointed and resourced to ensure that they can give proper attention to the workload.
277	Death certification	National guidance should set out standard methodologies for approaching the certification of the cause of death to ensure, so far as possible, that similar approaches are universal
278		It should be a routine part of an independent Medical Examiners' role to seek out and consider any serious untoward incidents or adverse incident reports relating to the deceased, to ensure that all circumstances are taken into account whether or not referred to in the medical records.
279		So far as is practicable, the responsibility for certifying the cause of death should be undertaken and fulfilled by the consultant, or another senior and fully qualified clinician in charge of a patient's case or treatment.
280	Appropriate and sensitive contact with bereaved families	Both the bereaved family and the certifying doctor should be asked whether they have any concerns about the death or the circumstances surrounding it, and guidance should be given to hospital staff encouraging them to raise any concerns they may have with the independent Medical Examiner.
281		It is important that independent Medical Examiners and any others having to approach families for this purpose have careful training in how to undertake this sensitive task in a manner least likely to cause additional and unnecessary distress.

including the deaths of mothers and babies, concluded: '*It is our view that the possibility of outlying behaviour such as this requires a failsafe system that would provide early warning of such problems by scrutinising the pattern of deaths of both mothers and babies . . . a mechanism already in use in other countries has been put forward to scrutinise all deaths in this way that would, by its nature, pick up maternal and neonatal deaths. This is the appointment of medical examiners, initially proposed by Dame Janet Smith as a recommendation of the Shipman Inquiry, subsequently endorsed by the Luce review, put into enabling legislation in 2009 but not yet implemented. It is our view that implementing these proposals should be reactivated as the best means to provide the necessary scrutiny, not just of maternity-related deaths, but of all deaths*'.[15]

The Department of Health[16] published a Consultation (Introduction of Medical Examiners and Reforms to Death Certification in England and Wales: Policy and Draft Regulations). The intended benefits of the new Medical Examiner system to the public, health service and local authorities are listed in Table 1.3.

After the 2016 Consultation, an inquiry into the Gosport War Memorial Hospital[17] found that the lives of more than 450 patients were shortened while in the hospital, despite concerns by families who had persistently raised questions about how their loved ones had been treated and similar concerns raised by nurses about prescribing practices of opiate medicine.

Table 1.3 Intended benefits of the introduction of the Medical Examiner service to England and Wales

o It will be fair – all deaths will be scrutinised in a robust, and proportionate way regardless of whether they are followed by burial or cremation;
o It will be independent – a Medical Examiner will scrutinise all medical certificates of cause of death (MCCD) prepared by the attending doctor;
o It will be transparent – families will have the cause of death explained to them, including clarification of medical terms, and be able to ask questions or raise concerns;
o It will be robust – there will be a protocol that recognises different levels of risk depending on the circumstances and stated cause of death;
o It will be accurate – the Medical Examiner will be an experienced doctor, capable of ensuring that the MCCD is completed fully and accurately, providing the NHS, the Office for National Statistics, local authorities and wide range of other users with better quality cause of death statistics to inform health policy, the planning and evaluation of health services and international comparisons;
o It will be efficient – it will help to make sure that the right cases are reported to Coroners; and
o It will improve safety – the new system will allow easier identification of trends, unusual patterns and local clinical governance issues and make malpractice easier to detect.

Source: Taken from Department of Health Introduction of Medical Examiners and Reforms to Death Certification in England & Wales: Policy and Draft Regulations, 2016.[16]

In June 2018, Jeremy Hunt (then Secretary of State for Health) announced the roll out of the appointment of Medical Examiners.[18] This implementation appears to have been finally precipitated by the case of Hadiza Bawa-Garba, a trainee paediatrician convicted of gross negligence manslaughter and struck off following the death of Jack Adcock, a child in her care. The Medical Practitioners Tribunal Service suspended Dr Bawa-Garba for 12 months on 13 June 2017. The General Medical Council successfully appealed, and Dr Bawa-Garba was struck off the medical register on 25 January 2018. On 13 August 2018, Dr Bawa-Garba won an appeal against being struck off, restoring the one-year suspension. Many healthcare professionals have raised concerns that Dr Bawa-Garba was being unduly punished for failings in the system, notably the understaffing on the day. Linked to this, was Sir Norman Williams' report, Gross Negligence Manslaughter in Healthcare. The report[19] was instigated to consider the wider patient-safety impact resulting from concerns among healthcare professionals that simple errors could result in prosecution for gross negligence manslaughter, even if they occur in the context of broader organisational and system failings. Amongst other recommendations, the Williams Report noted: '*The Government is introducing a system in England and Wales, where all non-coronial deaths are subject to a Medical Examiner's scrutiny. The introduction of Medical Examiners is designed to deliver a more comprehensive system of assurance for all non-coronial deaths. While not specifically concerned with gross negligence manslaughter, the introduction of Medical Examiners aims to improve the quality and appropriateness of referrals of deaths to Coroners and to increase transparency for the bereaved and offer them an opportunity to raise any concerns. The panel supports this aim and the introduction of Medical Examiners.*'[19]

Thus, from April 2019 a national system of MEs was introduced to acute NHS trusts (and some specialist trusts) in England, and by NHS Wales Shared Services Partnership (NWSSP) in Wales. These Medical Examiner services would be provided by Medical Examiner offices based within a (predominantly) hospital setting both in England and in Wales. It is fair to say that this action, to provide support for bereaved families and to improve patient safety, has to be considered a direct response to the repeated and (in some cases) historic recommendations in reports and public inquiries. And although Shipman, Mid Staffordshire and Morecambe Bay were the key drivers, there were other examples of concerns being raised by families and/or healthcare professional whistleblowers and being repeatedly ignored. For example, similar concerns were reported in the final Ockenden Report published in 2022 which identified failures to investigate, to learn and to improve within an NHS maternity service. The Ockenden Report investigated allegations of poor care after bereaved families had raised concerns where babies andmothers died or potentially suffered significant harm whilst receiving maternity care at The Shrewsbury and Telford Hospital NHS Trust.[20]

It will be noted that as the ME system was being established in 2019/2020, barely nine months into this development, health services were suddenly facing unprecedented pressures caused by the coronavirus pandemic. In response to the pandemic, the Coronavirus Act 2020 provided easements to facilitate the certification of deaths and reduce the administrative burden on overstretched doctors. Despite the massively increased workload, and the option of pausing development, many Medical Examiner services opted to progress throughout and played an important role in the pandemic response in a variety of ways, including supporting frontline clinicians in writing MCCDs or becoming full-time certifiers, releasing frontline doctors from an administrative task so that they could prioritise frontline caring duties. In part, this was driven by the consideration that at times of pressure, more clinical mistakes or errors might be made, and this was exactly the time when competent and independent oversight was required. Another important benefit was that interacting with a Medical Examiner gave bereaved families the opportunity to ask questions and understand what happened to their loved one during their final illness, at a time when most hospital visiting was suspended. Guidance was issued by NHS England and NHS Improvement about the Coronavirus Act easements, which simplified and streamlined many death certification functions and enabled ME offices to continue to develop, even if they were not staffed to the proposed level outlined in the national model by the National Medical Examiner.[21] If anything, the coronavirus pandemic made the need for the development of the ME system even more relevant.[22]

There remain a number of unresolved issues about the remit of the Medical Examiner. Stillbirths are currently not considered within the role of scrutiny, but many concerns relate to maternity and perinatal deaths. The findings and recommendations of a consultation in the UK by HM Government[23] on coronial investigations of stillbirths are still awaited. It is possible that the remit of Coroners and MEs will be extended to cover stillbirths at some point, particularly if the death occurs at full term or during labour. Meanwhile, hospital scandals (where whistleblowers' and families' concerns have been ignored) continue to arise, for example in Nottingham.[24] It would be a major concern if such a scandal arose in a hospital with an established Medical Examiner Service, purely because such deaths were considered not to be part of the MEs' remit.

Conclusions

Despite almost two decades of delays and some change in form, a new, independent Medical Examiner system has been introduced in England and Wales and is likely to be the most significant advance in the independent medicolegal investigation of death within living memory. Scandals and poor care continue to be identified from hospitals prior to the introduction of MEs. Paradoxically, although the drivers for its introduction were, in part, community and neonatal/child/maternity deaths, these were not the first patient groups to be subject to Medical Examiner scrutiny.

For pragmatic reasons, adult, in-hospital deaths were the first cohort of deaths where the system could be introduced, and since 2019, despite a pandemic, the Medical Examiner system has advanced and developed. Although safeguards to provide independence are present (with an additional reporting structure outside the acute hospital management structure), those outside the system may perceive that there is the possibility of lack of independence. This remains one of the challenges for Medical Examiner services – to be recognised as truly independent. It is likely that, in 2023, all non-coronial deaths in England and Wales (~400000 per annum) in hospitals and the community will be subject to ME scrutiny. At this stage, it is unclear whether the system will achieve one of its stated aims, namely, '[allowing] *easier identification of trends, unusual patterns and local clinical governance issues and* [making] *malpractice easier to detect'* but as the system progresses, there is optimism that this will be achieved, and will be a model for other jurisdictions to follow. Whether the ME system can identify and prevent future scandals about patient safety and care is the big unknown and, if it can, it will have been worth the wait.

REFERENCES

1. Office for National Statistics. Deaths Registered in England & Wales, 2020. https://www.ons. gov.uk/peoplepopulationandcommunity/birthsdeathsandmarriages/deaths/datasets/death sregisteredinenglandandwalesseriesdrreferencetables (accessed 17 December 2021).
2. Ministry of Justice. Coroner Statistics Annual 2019, England and Wales, 2020. https://assets. publishing.service.gov.uk/government/uploads/system/uploads/attachment_data/file/888314/ Coroners_Statistics_Annual_2019_.pdf (accessed 17 December 2021).
3. Department of Health and Social Care. Medical Examiners: Statement made on 9 June 2022. Statement UIN HCWS85. https://questions-statements.parliament.uk/written-statements/ detail/2022-06-09/hcws85 (accessed 22 June 2022)
4. House of Commons Constitutional Affairs Committee. Reform of the Coroners' System and Death Certification. Eighth Report of Session 2005–2006. https://publications.parliament.uk/ pa/cm200506/cmselect/cmconst/902/902i.pdf (accessed 17 December 2021).

5. Home Office/Department of Health. Learning from Tragedy, Keeping Patients Safe. Overview of the Government's action programme in response to the recommendations of the Shipman Inquiry, 2007. https://assets.publishing.service.gov.uk/government/uploads/system/uploads/attachment_data/file/228886/7014.pdf (accessed 17 December 2021).

6. Ministry of Justice. Medical Practitioners: Guidance on completing cremation forms, 2012. https://www.gov.uk/government/publications/medical-practitioners-guidance-on-completing-cremation-forms (accessed 17 December 2021).

7. Home Office/Department of Health. The Shipman Enquiry. Third report. Death certification and investigation of deaths by coroners, 2003. https://assets.publishing.service.gov.uk/government/uploads/system/uploads/attachment_data/file/273227/5854.pdf (accessed 17 December 2021).

8. Coroners and Justice Act 2009. https://www.legislation.gov.uk/ukpga/2009/25/data.pdf (accessed 17 December 2021).

9. Department of Health. Consultation on improving the process of death certification, 2007. [ARCHIVED CONTENT] Consultation on Improving the Process of Death Certification: Department of Health – Consultations (nationalarchives.gov.uk)

10. Luce T, Hodder E, McAuley D. Death Certification and Investigation in England, Wales and Northern Ireland: The report of a fundamental review 2003 ('the Luce Review'), 2004. https://www.semanticscholar.org/paper/Death-Certification-and-Investigation-in-England%2C-a-Luce-Hodder/51b2d4ff17e9a4a1bcf34557b34d1e9ae717cf14 (accessed 17 December 2021).

11. Department for Constitutional Affairs. Coroner Reform: The Government's Draft Bill. Improving death investigation in England and Wales. London: Stationery Office, 2006. https://assets.publishing.service.gov.uk/government/uploads/system/uploads/attachment_data/file/272304/6849.pdf (accessed 17 December 2021).

12. Baker R, Cordner S. Reform of Investigation of Deaths. A draft bill on the coroner system misses important chances. *BMJ* 2006; 333: 107–108.

13. Department of Health Lead Regional Director for Death Certification Reforms (2012). https://assets.publishing.service.gov.uk/government/uploads/system/uploads/attachment_data/file/215446/dh_129887.pdf

14. Francis R. Report of the Mid Staffordshire NHS Foundation Trust Public Inquiry, 2013. https://www.gov.uk/government/publications/report-of-the-mid-staffordshire-nhs-foundation-trust-public-inquiry (accessed 17 December 2021).

15. Kirkup B. The Report of the Morecambe Bay Investigation, 2015. https://assets.publishing.service.gov.uk/government/uploads/system/uploads/attachment_data/file/408480/47487_MBI_Accessible_v0.1.pdf (accessed 17 December 2021).

16. Department of Health. Introduction of Medical Examiners and Reforms to Death Certification in England and Wales: Policy and Draft Regulations, 2016. https://assets.publishing.service.gov.uk/government/uploads/system/uploads/attachment_data/file/517184/DCR_Consultion_Document.pdf (accessed 17 December 2021).

17. Gosport War Memorial Hospital. The Report of the Gosport Independent Panel, 2018. https://www.gosportpanel.independent.gov.uk/panel-report/ (accessed 17 December 2021).

18. Laville S. NHS patient deaths to be investigated by medical examiners, *The Guardian* 11 June 2018. https://www.theguardian.com/society/2018/jun/11/nhs-patient-deaths-investigated-medical-examiners-jeremy-hunt (accessed 17 December 2021).

19. Williams N. Gross Negligence Manslaughter in Healthcare. The report of a rapid policy review ('the Williams Report'), 2018. https://assets.publishing.service.gov.uk/government/uploads/system/uploads/attachment_data/file/717946/Williams_Report.pdf (accessed 17 December 2021).

20. Ockenden D. Findings, conclusions and essential actions from the independent review of maternity services at The Shrewsbury and Telford Hospital NHS Trust published 30 March 2022. https://assets.publishing.service.gov.uk/government/uploads/system/uploads/attachment_data/file/1064302/Final-Ockenden-Report-web-accessible.pdf (accessed 12 May 2022).

21. National Medical Examiner for England and Wales. National Medical Examiner's Report *2020*. https://www.england.nhs.uk/wp-content/uploads/2021/04/B0413_NME-Report-2020-FINAL.pdf (accessed 17 December 2021).

22. NHS England and NHS Improvement. Coronavirus Act – Excess Death Provisions: Information and guidance for medical practitioners, 2020. https://www.england.nhs.uk/coronavirus/wp-content/uploads/sites/52/2020/03/COVID-19-Act-excess-death-provisions-info-and-guidance-31-03-20.pdf (accessed 17 December 2021).

23. Lord Chancellor and Secretary of State for Justice. Consultation on Coronial Investigations of Stillbirths, 2019. https://consult.justice.gov.uk/digital-communications/coronial-investigations-of-stillbirths/supporting_documents/Consultation%20on%20coronial%20investigations%20of%20stillbirths%20web.pdf (accessed 17 December 2021).

24. Lintern S. Revealed: Dozens of baby deaths after errors at one of UK's largest hospitals, *Independent,* 30 June 2021. https://www.independent.co.uk/news/health/nottingham-hospitals-maternity-baby-deaths-b1874132.html (accessed 17 December 2021).

CHAPTER 2

The Medical Examiner Service in England and Wales: Structure

Jason Payne-James, Suzy Lishman and Jason Shannon

Introduction

The introduction of a national Medical Examiner system for the medicolegal review of non-coronial death was rolled out from April 2019 in England and Wales after a prolonged period of gestation (see Chapter 1). The broad principles for the introduction were the same for both England and Wales, but because of the differences in NHS structure in the two countries there are differences in how services have developed. This chapter summarises the structure and function of the Medical Examiner Service, have been put into practice in both countries. As the Medical Examiner system is developing in part from the ground up, based on broad principles provided by the National Medical Examiner (NME), there is some variation in how each service functions. This chapter outlines how a Medical Examiner Service (MES) works in England and Wales.

Structure and Function of the Medical Examiner Service in England

The Medical Examiner system introduced in 2019 aims to:

- provide bereaved families with greater transparency and opportunities to raise concerns
- improve the quality/accuracy of medical certification of cause of death
- ensure referrals to Coroners are appropriate
- support local learning/improvement by identifying matters in need of clinical governance and related processes
- provide the public with greater safeguards through improved and consistent scrutiny of all non-coronial deaths, and support healthcare providers to improve care through better learning
- align with related systems such as the National Learning from Deaths Framework and Universal Mortality Reviews.

Medical Examiners (MEs), supported by Medical Examiner Officers (MEOs), scrutinise (review) all deaths that do not fall under HM Coroner's jurisdiction across a local area. MEs are trained, independent, senior doctors. Any practising, or recently retired, medical practitioner who has been fully registered for at least five years and has a licence to practise with the General Medical Council (GMC), can apply to be an ME but the NME advises that MEs should be consultant-grade doctors, other senior doctors from a range of disciplines or GPs with an equivalent level of experience. In the UK, the Royal College of Pathologists is the lead medical Royal College for MEs and is responsible for training MEs and MEOs. Training is currently a combination of e-learning and face-to-face, and successful completion permits ME or MEO membership of the Royal College of Pathologists. By December 2022, more than 1600 MEs had been trained by the Royal College of Pathologists. MEs and MEOs are employed in the NHS but have an additional, separate professional line of accountability to regional (*see* Chapter 3) and national ME teams. Independence is overseen by the NME, supported by seven regional teams of Regional Medical Examiners and Regional Medical Examiner Officers.

The role of the NME is to provide professional and strategic leadership to the Regional Medical Examiner teams (in England) and Lead Medical Examiner for Wales. In England, Regional MEs support a network of ME offices in acute hospital trusts. Most trusts have a Lead ME and a number of other MEs who may come from a range of different medical specialties.

MEs generally work part-time, typically one or two four-hour sessions per week. The NME supports safeguards for public, patient-safety monitoring and informs the national learning from deaths agenda, and produces an annual report.[1]

Current guidance suggests that in order to provide adequate cover to scrutinise 100% of deaths, one whole-time equivalent ME and three whole-time MEOs will be required for every 3000 deaths.[1] These figures have been determined from pilot studies that have been in place since about 2008. As the MES is still in the adolescent stage of development, it is likely that these figures will be refined, as the availability and expertise of the MES becomes more widely recognised, and its role expands.

The initial introductory phase of ME Services has been in acute hospital trusts in England and across health boards in Wales. All were asked to set up (starting in April 2019) ME offices focussing on deaths within their own organisation on a non-statutory basis. Initially, adult deaths were the priority, with only some MES teams reviewing neonatal and child deaths. In an ambitious plan, it is intended that every non-coronial death in England and Wales will be scrutinised by MEs when the system becomes statutory (anticipated to be in 2023). Some ME services are on track to achieve this, but not all are yet achieving 100% scrutiny of hospital deaths, let alone those in the community. For practical reasons, the MES teams in hospital will also predominantly act as the hubs for scrutiny of community deaths (e.g. at home, in nursing homes, hospices or community hospitals). There are a number of challenges involved in this roll-out into the community, not least multiple electronic notes systems, varying IT governance issues, including access to community medical records and communicating with healthcare professionals in the community (*see* Chapter 12). However, a number of multidisciplinary working pilot studies are beginning to make progress with this. In June 2021, NHS England and NHS Improvement confirmed what local health systems need to do to implement the NME system for scrutiny of non-coronial deaths across all health settings. This information has been provided to GPs, clinical commissioning groups, integrated care systems and chief executive officers of foundation and NHS trusts and gives intended timelines of MES progression to provide ME scrutiny of non-coronial deaths across all non-acute sectors perhaps by the end of 2022.[2]

On 28 April 2022, the Health and Care Act received Royal Assent, which will provide the mechanism to place the role of the Medical Examiner on a statutory footing (via secondary legislation) in 2023.

Medical Examiners

MEs are trained in the legal and clinical elements of death certification processes. MEs are senior doctors who, in the immediate period before the death is registered (within five days), independently scrutinise the causes of death. In all cases not investigated by HM Coroner, the ME addresses the following issues:

- What did the person die from? (ensuring accuracy of cause of death on the Medical Certificate of Cause of Death [MCCD])
- Does this case need to be reported to a Coroner? (ensuring timely, accurate referral)
- Are there any clinical governance concerns? (ensuring the relevant authority is notified).

To achieve this, MEs complete the following steps to arrive at their decision:

- speak to the doctor who was treating the patient on their final illness (the qualified attending practitioner – QAP) to discuss the proposed MCCD and enquire about any concerns of care
- review the medical records and any supporting diagnostic information
- agree the proposed cause of death and the overall accuracy of the MCCD with the QAP
- discuss the cause of death with the next of kin/informant and establish if they have any concerns with care.

Further roles that the MEs provide include:

- acting as a medical advice resource for HM Coroner
- acting as a medical advice resource for registration services

- acting as a medical advice resource for organ donation teams
- initiating escalations for deaths where learning might be gained (e.g. structured judgement reviews, serious untoward incident investigations)
- ensuring that patterns or concerns about care by clinicians and others are raised appropriately
- feeding back praise or compliments to individuals and teams.

As the national ME system develops and there is greater awareness amongst other health professionals and those whose role includes support and management of the deceased and bereaved, an ME may be asked questions about matters not directly within their primary roles, for example, organ donation, genetic testing, post mortems or funeral arrangements. The ME needs to be able to direct such queries to appropriate teams. It is also important to recognise that the ME system is intended to flag and identify concerns about care before death, but not to investigate such concerns. Unsurprisingly, there is no clear line between making adequate enquiry to determine whether something needs escalation, and investigation itself. As with HM Coroners, and their decision-making, there is substantial variability in how different MEs might approach a case and that might, in turn, be influenced by the stance of the local Coroner. Interpretation of the notification requirements for deaths to Coroners[4] is an art rather than a science and a local example of a chart to assist clinical teams in knowing when to notify is provided in Figure 2.1. However, most Coroners will now require a clinical team to have discussed any cases with the MES before notification is commenced.

Once an MES is up and running, it will rapidly become a source of advice for HM Coroner, registration services and organ-donation teams. It is essential that each MES devotes adequate time to education and training as, despite considerable time having passed since MEs were introduced, there is still a lack of widespread understanding of the nature and role of the ME system. It is vital for those healthcare professionals in contact with MEs to realise that MEs and MEOs often identify praise and compliments about teams, individuals and hospitals and disseminating that praise to those individuals and teams is another very important part of the role. Most MEs are likely to find that praise about care of a patient before death considerably outweighs criticism.

The MES will need to liaise locally with mortality governance systems teams (*see* Chapter 11), and this may provide an opportunity to develop electronic versions of documents, pending the introduction of a national ME software system.

Medical Examiner Officers

Medical Examiner Officers (MEOs) are the golden thread or glue that provides the continuity between (mostly part-time) MEs and all other parties involved in the care of the deceased and bereaved. Their relationship to MEs can be equated to that of Coroners' officers and Coroners. They perform many of the functions

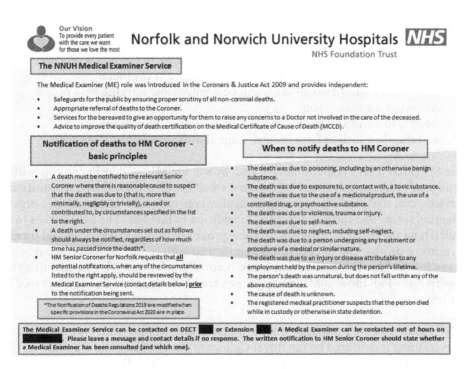

Our Vision
To provide every patient
with the care we want
for those we love the most

Norfolk and Norwich University Hospitals NHS

NHS Foundation Trust

The NNUH Medical Examiner Service

The Medical Examiner (ME) role was introduced in the Coroners & Justice Act 2009 and provides independent:

- Safeguards for the public by ensuring proper scrutiny of all non-coronial deaths.
- Appropriate referral of deaths to the Coroner.
- Services for the bereaved to give an opportunity for them to raise any concerns to a Doctor not involved in the care of the deceased.
- Advice to improve the quality of death certification on the Medical Certificate of Cause of Death (MCCD).

Notification of deaths to HM Coroner - basic principles

- A death must be notified to the relevant Senior Coroner where there is reasonable cause to suspect that the death was due to (that is, more than minimally, negligibly or trivially), caused or contributed to, by circumstances specified in the list to the right.
- A death under the circumstances set out as follows should always be notified, regardless of how much time has passed since the death*.
- HM Senior Coroner for Norfolk requests that **all** potential notifications, when any of the circumstances listed to the right apply, should be reviewed by the Medical Examiner Service (contact details below) **prior** to the notification being sent.

*The Notification of Deaths Regulations 2019 are modified when specific provisions in the Coronavirus Act 2020 are in place.

When to notify deaths to HM Coroner

- The death was due to poisoning, including by an otherwise benign substance.
- The death was due to exposure to, or contact with, a toxic substance.
- The death was due to the use of a medicinal product, the use of a controlled drug, or psychoactive substance.
- The death was due to violence, trauma or injury.
- The death was due to self-harm.
- The death was due to neglect, including self-neglect.
- The death was due to a person undergoing any treatment or procedure of a medical or similar nature.
- The death was due to an injury or disease attributable to any employment held by the person during the person's lifetime.
- The person's death was unnatural, but does not fall within any of the above circumstances.
- The cause of death is unknown.
- The registered medical practitioner suspects that the person died while in custody or otherwise in state detention.

The Medical Examiner Service can be contacted on DECT ▇▇ or Extension ▇▇. A Medical Examiner can be contacted out of hours on ▇▇▇▇. Please leave a message and contact details if no response. The written notification to HM Senior Coroner should state whether a Medical Examiner has been consulted (and which one).

Figure 2.1 Basic principles of notification to HM Coroner [adapted from Notification of Deaths Regulations 2019 guidance] and utilised at the Norfolk and Norwich University Hospitals NHS Foundation Trust.

of the ME, via delegated authority. MEOs manage the Medical Examiner Service in their hospital and in Wales are located full time in the hub sites. Currently some MEOs in England fulfil other functions (e.g. bereavement advisor) but, realistically, it is appropriate that the role is undertaken full-time.

MEOs cannot perform scrutiny of the medical records of deceased patients but may undertake a preliminary screening of those records, support and assist the MEs, and make contact with QAPs and bereaved families. The extent of their involvement (and thus what tasks can be undertaken via delegated authority) may depend on their previous clinical and other experience and should be agreed locally with their Lead MEOs and MEs. MEOs come from a wide range of backgrounds, including nursing, bereavement and mortuary. The broader the range of backgrounds of the Medical Examiner Service team, the better the MES can meet the needs of other stakeholders. Those appointed to MEO roles (whether with a clinical background or not) should encompass the following (non-exhaustive) skills and competences:

- previously have experience in a patient- or customer-facing role and of working in either current death certification systems, or a clinical or NHS setting

- have an understanding of medical records and disease pathology
- be able to provide advice on terminology and causes of death, and to explain these and the ME's thoughts and rationale to Coroner's officers, doctors and those with no medical or healthcare background
- have strong interpersonal skills and be comfortable working with people following a bereavement
- be able to build and maintain effective relationships with other stakeholders such as faith groups, funeral directors and legal services.

The MEO has a very responsible role and, as will the ME, will be interacting with a range of professionals including doctors, allied health professionals, registration services, coronial services, crematoria, medical referees, faith organisations, organ donation teams and funeral directors, in addition to families. The MEO needs to understand the respective roles of all these groups to ensure expeditious and timely scrutiny of deaths, and to keep families informed with sensitivity and compassion. Many roles within these groups and stakeholders overlap and it is essential that the sensitivities of all those contributing to the care of the deceased and the bereaved are respected.

MEOs undergo core training and face-to-face training in the same way as MEs. This training is delivered by the Royal College of Pathologists, and training continued (remotely and successfully) throughout the COVID-19 pandemic.

How Does a Medical Examiner Service Work?

Every MES will have different local processes and protocols to best service the needs of their host organisation, whilst running an effective scrutiny process. MEs, MEOs and the MES are responsible for the scrutiny of every death within a hospital and will also be responsible for scrutiny of every out-of-hospital death in the future. In order to achieve the aspirational target of 100% of deaths being scrutinised within 24 hours of a death, adequate personnel and resources are required. The ME system is, to some extent, being developed from the ground up, using principles established by the NME office.

As the MES is undertaking contact with clinicians and others, such as families, it is essential that there is documentary evidence of any contact, to enable review of decision-making and assist in further investigations. Two main documents are common to most ME offices, the ME-1A and ME-1B forms (Figures 2.2, 2.3a and 2.3b). These may be locally adapted. Form ME-1A (not always used) predominantly contains basic administrative data. This form may not always be used in hospitals but may be more useful for remote working, and for assisting with community deaths. Form ME-1B provides information about the scrutiny undertaken by the ME Service including the date and time of the deceased's death, the ME review of notes, the sources of information used, any discussions with the QAP, HM Coroner and the family, and any record of escalation. It also records the outcomes of these discussions, including any modification to the MCCD. It is an important record that summarises the entire scrutiny process and may be discoverable in any litigation.

Once the MES has been informed of a death, the MEO (under delegated authority) may, if suitably competent, undertake a pre-review of the deceased's medical records, contact the QAP to determine what is proposed for the MCCD and identify any concerns. These will then be discussed with the ME, who may make their own further enquiries having fully scrutinised the deceased's last medical admission. Sometimes (e.g. if there is lack of clarity about previous employment and the patient has died with a possible employment-related condition such as pulmonary fibrosis) further review of historical medical notes and discussion with the clinical team will be required. Scrutiny should always be proportionate. It is not expected to be a detailed forensic analysis. Once the MCCD wording is agreed with the QAP (suggestions on the wording or formulation of the MCCD are only advisory, but rarely ignored) then the bereaved family can be contacted for their comments. There are three specific elements that are important when speaking to the bereaved. These are: offering condolences; asking whether there were any concerns about their relative's care; and explaining the wording on the MCCD. The wording on the MCCD is also subject to review by the local registration

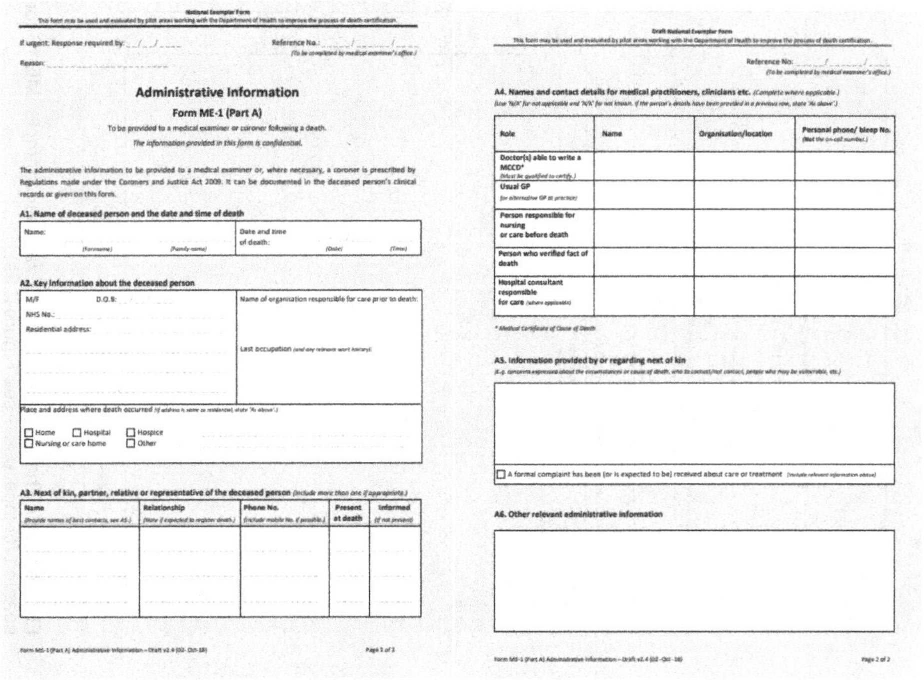

National Exemplar Form

This form may be used and evaluated by pilot areas working with the Department of Health to improve the process of death certification.

If urgent: Response required by: __/__/____

Reference No.: ____/____/____
(To be completed by medical examiner's office.)

Reason: ____________

Administrative Information

Form ME-1 (Part A)

To be provided to a medical examiner or coroner following a death.

The information provided in this form is confidential.

The administrative information to be provided to a medical examiner or, where necessary, a coroner is prescribed by Regulations made under the Coroners and Justice Act 2009. It can be documented in the deceased person's clinical records or given on this form.

A1. Name of deceased person and the date and time of death

Name: (Forename) (Family name)	Date and time of death: (Date) (Time)

A2. Key information about the deceased person

M/F D.O.B: NHS No.: Residential address:	Name of organisation responsible for care prior to death: Last occupation (and any relevant work history)
Place and address where death occurred (If address is same as residential, state 'As above'.) ☐ Home ☐ Hospital ☐ Hospice ☐ Nursing or care home ☐ Other	

A3. Next of kin, partner, relative or representative of the deceased person (Include more than one if appropriate.)

Name (Provide names of best contacts, see A5.)	Relationship (Note if expected to register death.)	Phone No. (Include mobile No. if possible.)	Present at death	Informed (if not present)

Form ME-1 (Part A) Administrative Information – Draft v2.4 (02-Oct-18) Page 1 of 2

Draft National Exemplar Form

This form may be used and evaluated by pilot areas working with the Department of Health to improve the process of death certification.

Reference No: ____/____/____
(To be completed by medical examiner's office.)

A4. Names and contact details for medical practitioners, clinicians etc. (Complete where applicable.)

Role	Name	Organisation/location	Personal phone/ bleep No. (Not the on-call number.)
Doctor(s) able to write a MCCD* (Must be qualified to certify.)			
Usual GP (or alternative GP at practice)			
Person responsible for nursing or care before death			
Person who verified fact of death			
Hospital consultant responsible for care (where applicable)			

* Medical Certificate of Cause of Death

A5. Information provided by or regarding next of kin

☐ A formal complaint has been (or is expected to be) received about care or treatment (Include relevant information above)

A6. Other relevant administrative information

Form ME-1 (Part A) Administrative Information – Draft v2.4 (02-Oct-18) Page 2 of 2

Figure 2.2 The National Medical Examiner exemplar ME-1A form (may not always be used or adapted for local use).

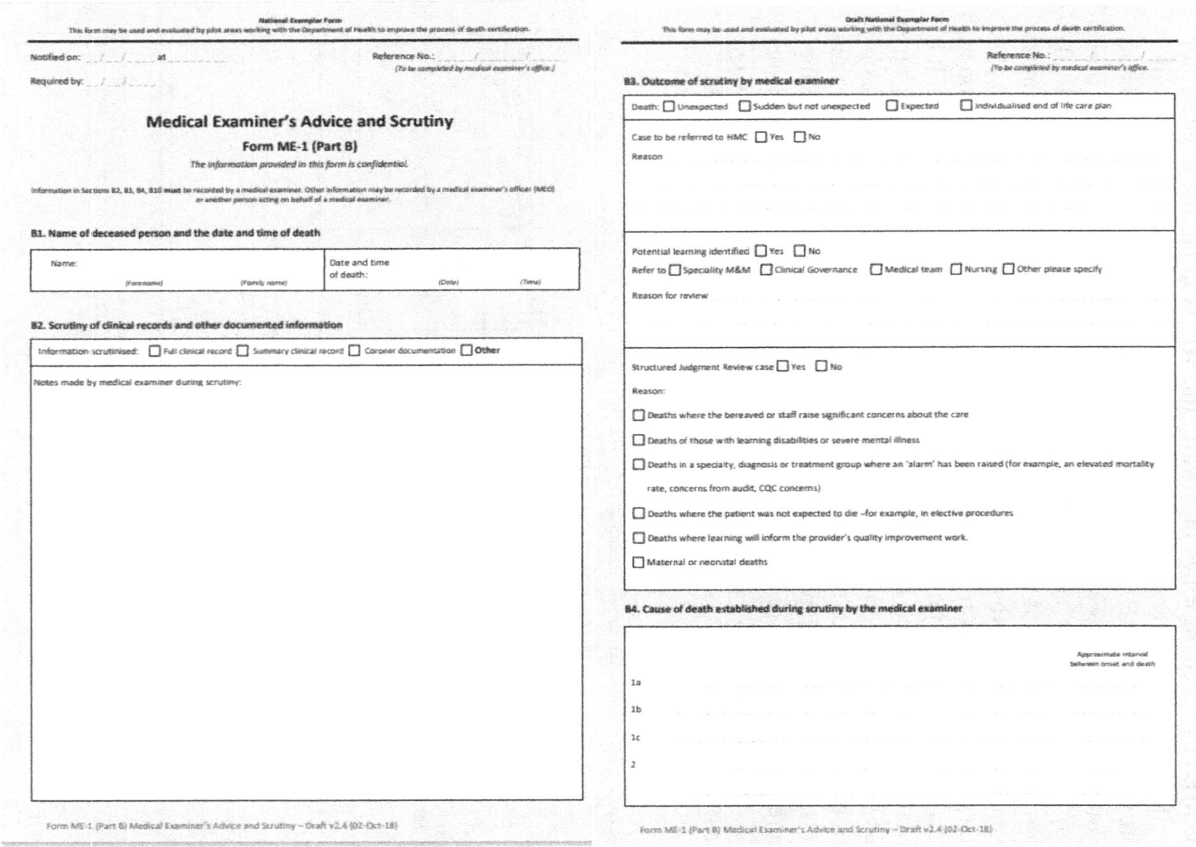

National Exemplar Form
This form may be used and evaluated by pilot areas working with the Department of Health to improve the process of death certification.

Notified on: __/__/____ at ________ Reference No.: ____/____/____
(To be completed by medical examiner's office.)

Required by: __/__/____

Medical Examiner's Advice and Scrutiny

Form ME-1 (Part B)

The information provided in this form is confidential.

Information in Sections B2, B3, B4, B10 must be recorded by a medical examiner. Other information may be recorded by a medical examiner's officer (MEO) or another person acting on behalf of a medical examiner.

B1. Name of deceased person and the date and time of death

Name: (Forename) (Family name)	Date and time of death: (Date) (Time)

B2. Scrutiny of clinical records and other documented information

Information scrutinised: ☐ Full clinical record ☐ Summary clinical record ☐ Coroner documentation ☐ Other

Notes made by medical examiner during scrutiny:

Form ME-1 (Part B) Medical Examiner's Advice and Scrutiny – Draft v2.4 (02-Oct-18)

Draft National Exemplar Form
This form may be used and evaluated by pilot areas working with the Department of Health to improve the process of death certification.

Reference No.: ____/____/____
(To be completed by medical examiner's office.

B3. Outcome of scrutiny by medical examiner

Death: ☐ Unexpected ☐ Sudden but not unexpected ☐ Expected ☐ Individualised end of life care plan

Case to be referred to HMC ☐ Yes ☐ No
Reason

Potential learning identified ☐ Yes ☐ No
Refer to ☐ Speciality M&M ☐ Clinical Governance ☐ Medical team ☐ Nursing ☐ Other please specify
Reason for review

Structured Judgment Review case ☐ Yes ☐ No
Reason:
☐ Deaths where the bereaved or staff raise significant concerns about the care
☐ Deaths of those with learning disabilities or severe mental illness
☐ Deaths in a specialty, diagnosis or treatment group where an 'alarm' has been raised (for example, an elevated mortality rate, concerns from audit, CQC concerns)
☐ Deaths where the patient was not expected to die –for example, in elective procedures
☐ Deaths where learning will inform the provider's quality improvement work.
☐ Maternal or neonatal deaths

B4. Cause of death established during scrutiny by the medical examiner

Approximate interval between onset and death

1a
1b
1c
2

Form ME-1 (Part B) Medical Examiner's Advice and Scrutiny – Draft v2.4 (02-Oct-18)

Figure 2.3a The National Medical Examiner exemplar ME-1B form (may not always be used or adapted for local use – see Figure 2.3b).

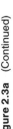

Figure 2.3a (Continued)

ME-1B NNUH v10 3 7 2020   Reference No: NNUH

ME Advice and Scrutiny Form ME-1 (Part B)

ME-1A & 1B are confidential and are only available for authorised use by, or on behalf of, the Medical Examiner Service & HM Coroner Service

Given name	Family Name	Date & Time of death:

Information Scrutinised: ☐ MCCD ☐ Medical records ☐ Summary Medical Record ☐ Other (noted below)

Documented cause of death available before scrutiny? ☐ Yes on ME-1A (if utilised) ☐ Yes on MCCD ☐ Yes Cremation 4 ☐ No

MEO Review of Notes:

Burial ☐   Cremation ☐
Under 18 ☐
Community Death (Hospital) ☐
Community Death (Other) ☐

(Note name of MEO and date of review and any contact with family or others)
_____

ME Scrutiny of Notes:

Death was: ☐ Unexpected   ☐ Sudden but not unexpected   ☐ Expected   ☐ Individual Plan of Care

---

☐   Proposed / certified causes of death documented on ME-1A or suggested by QAP before scrutiny accepted without change
☐   Cause(s) of death established during Medical Examiner scrutiny (and documented below)

1a)
1b)
1c)
2)

☐ ME-1A Completed   ☐ ME-1A Not Completed
QAP discussed with: ☐ Medical Examiner : ☐ Medical Examiner Officer (Name and Date)_____
QAP Name and Contact: _____
Summary of discussion with QAP doctor (if required)::

☐   Proposed / certified causes of death documented before scrutiny (or noted above) accepted without change
☐   Causes established by the Medical Examiner during scrutiny and agreed as documented below

1a)
1b)
1c)
2)

Figure 2.3b   Locally adapted ME-1B form (currently in use at the Norfolk and Norwich University Hospitals NHS Trust, Norwich, UK and integrated into the local mortality governance system).

Outcome of scrutiny

☐ No concerns identified by MES, healthcare professional or bereaved - MCCD not changed from QAP proposal

☐ Coroner has agreed to open an investigation and an MCCD is not required HM Coroner Reference Number: CR_____

☐ QAP has certified (or will certify) the death using causes agreed / revised during scrutiny

☐ Escalation - see below

Discussion with HM Coroner / HM Coroner's office *(if required during or after scrutiny):*

☐ Coroner does not need to investigate the death and has issued an HMC-1

Discussion with Family Member/Next of Kin/Other: *(name, status & contact details)*_____

Discussed by Medical Examiner/Medical Examiner Officer *(date)* _____ at *(time)* _____

Record time(s) and date(s) of any failed contact with NoK:_____

Condolences offered: ☐

Concerns about care:_____

_____

MCCD Content discussed: _____

Other matters arising (separate sheet if
required):_____

Outcome (eg referral to SJR, LG, HM Coroner), praise to individual or teams)

Escalation or Referral of Cases:
Case to be referred to HM Coroner   ☐ Yes   ☐ No   ☐ Already referred – Reference No:_____
Reason for referral:

Potential learning identified   ☐ Yes   ☐ No
Refer to ☐ Local Governance   ☐ DATIX ☐ Other please specify
Reason for review:

Structured Judgment Review case ☐ Yes   ☐ No
Criteria:
☐ Deaths where the bereaved or staff raise significant concerns about the care
☐ Deaths of those with learning disabilities or severe mental illness
☐ Deaths in a specialty, diagnosis or treatment group where an 'alarm' has been raised (for example, an elevated mortality rate, concerns from audit, CQC co
☐ Deaths where the patient was not expected to die – for example, in elective procedures
☐ Deaths where learning will inform the provider's quality improvement work
☐ Homeless
☐ Maternal or neonatal deaths

Praise and other issues:_____

The Medical Examiner Service has carried out an independent and proportionate scrutiny of this death as required. The estimated
completion time (ME + MEO) for each part was (minutes) - 1 Review of notes:_____2 Discussion with QAP: _____
3 Contacting and discussion with Next of Kin:_____ 4 Completion of Cremation Form 5 & Viewing of Deceased: _____

Name of Medical Examiner Officer _____ Signature: _____ Date:_____

Name of Medical Examiner _____ Signature: _____ Date:_____

Figure 2.3b   (Continued)

team. When an informant (normally a relative) registers a death, the registrar will review the MCCD. The Royal College of Pathologists now publishes the Cause of Death List,[5] a document that is intended not to reflect every possible cause of death but to address those conditions that often result in discussion between the MCCD-writing doctor, registrar and HM Coroner. Should a registrar identify that a cause of death written on the MCCD is not an 'acceptable' cause (e.g. renal failure, with no underlying condition identified) then they would be required to notify that death to HM Coroner, and registration would be paused pending review. With an MES in place, such instances should be rare, as the MCCD will have been reviewed and discussed by the ME who will provide guidance as to appropriate completion. In some register office areas, registrars will accept a cause of death that is not on the 'acceptable' list, if the MCCD is countersigned by the Medical Examiner, confirming that it has been subject to scrutiny and there are no concerns. The Cause of Death List document also provides very useful advice on completion of MCCDs and for those informants registering deaths. The Notification of Deaths Regulations 2019, the Cause of Death List and a further publication, Guidance for Doctors Completing Medical Certificates of Cause of Death in England and Wales[6] are documents with which MEs and MEOs must be familiar to undertake their functions, and to appropriately advise others. These are sometimes modified (the latter being modified for the emergency period of the coronavirus pandemic and subsequently updated when the emergency Act expired) and so the MES needs to monitor any changes in guidance closely.

If concerns about care are raised, either by the bereaved or the QAP, it is for the MES to identify and escalate or, on some occasions, direct the family to a body, person or organisation most appropriate for their concerns. All of this should be documented in detail on the ME-1B. Under delegated authority, the MEOs can carry out many of the functions of the ME with the exception of the full review of the medical records and signing off the whole process (scrutiny) as complete. The outcome measures of importance at present are, the number of MCCDs where wording is changed; identifying concerns of next of kin; and ensuring appropriate notification to HM Coroner.

Structure and Function of the Medical Examiner Service in Wales

The Coroners and Justice Act 2009,[7] which places the ME system on a statutory footing, is not devolved and applies equally to Wales and England, although there are some devolved elements that apply to the terms and conditions for Medical Examiner appointment, fee setting and collection, which would come into force within a fully statutory system. NHS administration in Wales is entirely devolved to the Welsh Government and the Act, as applicable to Wales, indicated that Health Boards would host the service. In fact, in the non-statutory system, MEs are employed by NHS Wales Shared Services Partnership (NWSSP) and based in four hub offices, which are not linked to specific acute hospitals. The NHS in

Wales is based on an integrated care provider model with very little residual commissioning between organisations.

It was a joint determination by both the Welsh Government and the NHS care providers that the MES would sit within a separate and single organisation to strengthen and make explicit the independence of the Medical Examiner function but would also allow for economies of scale and flexibility of service delivery. NWSSP was chosen as the host organisation due to its primary function of delivering a range of largely non-clinical functions on behalf of NHS care providers.

The impact assessment from the pilot sites reflected in the Good Practice Guidance[1] sets out a baseline of one whole-time equivalent ME with three MEOs for the scrutiny of 3000 deaths. With an anticipated number of non-coronial deaths in Wales of around 30000, this made for a relatively straightforward calculation of the number of staff required once all deaths were required to be reviewed. However, these deaths are spread across several small- to medium-sized acute and non-acute hospital and community sites, reflecting the dispersed geography of Wales with a significant remote and rural population. The hosting arrangements, together with the changes associated with the Coronavirus Act 2020,[8, 9] which decoupled the requirement for viewing bodies and completing Cremation Form 5, allowed for a more centralised model of delivery from four hub sites based on non-hospital sites dealing with between 7000 to 10000 deaths rather than 1000–1500 deaths occurring in a typical hospital. Underpinning by a single governance framework and digital database has meant that the hub sites function identically, allowing an easy transfer of work across the whole of Wales within a single-managed and networked service. MEs, in particular, who often provide clinical services to hospitals and health boards, are able to be offered cases that the ME would not have had involvement in personally, and also that would not have been managed by the hospital or even the health board to which they have separate accountability as clinicians, thus fulfilling the requirements for independence set out in the recommendations of the Francis Report on the care failings in Mid-Staffordshire NHS Trust,[10] which stated that Medical Examiners should be independent of the organisation whose deaths they were scrutinising.

The principles of the MES are no different in Wales and, in particular, the aims of improving death certification, ensuring that the right deaths are referred to the Coroner and ensuring that the bereaved are provided with an opportunity to ask questions about the MCCD as well as raise any concerns they may have, are fundamentally embedded within the service and reflected in its configuration. The digital database has been designed to reflect this, to ensure that a signed ME-2 form (see Figure 2.4) indicates that the full processes of scrutiny have been undertaken, which will eventually serve as an authorisation of death registration in the statutory model. The database also permits detailed report generation for care providers to allow them to consider themes for triangulation with their wider quality improvement systems and an understanding of what their harm fingerprint might look like.

CORONERS AND JUSTICE ACT 2009

Form prescribed by the Death Certification Regulations 2016

Medical Examiner's Notification of Certified Cause of Death

This form notifies a registrar that a medical examiner has issued a Medical Certificate of Cause of Death with the MCCD number and cause shown below following referral of the death by a coroner. When this form has been fully completed, the registrar can use the medical examiner's certificate, pursuant to regulations under the Births and Deaths Registration Act 1953, to register the death and authorise burial or cremation.

Part A – Medical Examiner's Notification

Details of the deceased person:

Full forenames and family name: NHS No:

Age at death: Date of death

Place of death:

Certified cause of death: MCCD No.   issued after referral and receipt of *Coroner Form*

                                                                                                    Approximate interval

I (a)

  (b)

  (c)

  (d)

  (e) *(neonatal)*

II

Discussion of cause of death:

Name: Role: has discussed the cause of death with

Name: Relationship to deceased person:

The discussion took place on *(date)*   at *(time)*   and did not identify any concerns that required investigation by a coroner. The person named above has been advised that Part B of this form needs to be signed to confirm that the discussion has taken place and that a registrar cannot register the death or provide a certificate to authorise burial, cremation or other means of disposal until this signature has been provided.

Medical Examiner's declaration:

I hereby declare that I am a duly appointed medical examiner and that I have established and certified the cause of death stated above following independent scrutiny in accordance with the appropriate standards and procedures and that I am not aware of any matter that might cause a coroner to think that the death should be investigated. The information given on this form is true and accurate to the best of my knowledge and belief and I am aware that it is an offence if I knowingly and wilfully make a false statement.

Name: GMC No: Area:

Signature: Date:

Part B – Informant's confirmation *(to be completed at a Medical Examiner's Office or Register Office)*

Informant's name: Relationship to deceased:

I confirm that to the best of my knowledge and belief the discussion referred to above took place and provided an opportunity to raise any matters that might cause a coroner to think that the death should be investigated.

Signature: Provided at *(location)*:   Date:

Form ME-2(B) Medical Examiner's Notification of Certified Cause of Death   Page 1 of 1

Figure 2.4   The National Medical Examiner exemplar ME-2 form (may not always be used or adapted for local use).

Coroners in Wales were involved in the recruitment of Medical Examiners by sitting on the interview panels. There is a challenge in setting up a single service to run in partnership with seven separate Coroner jurisdictions, which has been alleviated, to some extent, by the requirement to withdraw local guidance to ensure greater consistency of death reporting under the Statutory Notification Regulations.[4] Further developments, in line with the recommendations from the Ministry of Justice Select Committee report, to consider a single Coroner service would be a welcome development for a single Medical Examiner Service such as the one that Wales has developed.

All deaths in Wales have been reviewed for much of the last decade following the recommendations of the Francis Report. It was always envisaged that the Stage 1 mortality review process developed as a result would be subsumed into the work of the Medical Examiner System when it was introduced. These independent processes overcome the challenges of variation in the quality of mortality review and allow collection and comparison of concerns. The independence of ME scrutiny is important for both the public and for care providers, as they can be assured that any concerns identified are not due to variation in the scrutiny process itself.[11]

MEs and MEOs are employed on a separate contract with NWSSP. Most MEs are working one or two sessions per week but as the service reaches maturity, the majority are planning to increase sessional commitments, which will assist with approaching the whole-time equivalent of 10 MEs in Wales. A further round of ME recruitment is planned to make up the shortfall. The MEOs typically work full time and a round of recruitment took place in July 2021. Most hospital deaths were being reviewed by September 2021.

Implementation has been supported by a comprehensive virtual CPD programme, often delivered by individuals within the service. The subjects presented are matched to the competency frameworks for staff, which are then evidenced either through the Agenda for Change PADR process for MEOs or the all-Wales Medical Appraisal and Revalidation System (MARS) for MEs in line with guidance from the Royal College of Pathologists referenced in the Good Practice Guidance.[1]

The roll out into the non-acute sector is potentially more straightforward owing to the difference in the configuration of the NHS in Wales described above. Some primary care providers and hospices have already been brought on board with data-sharing agreements in place. Shared services also hold the contracts for the GP records systems, creating the potential for a seamless access to primary care records for scrutiny. With nearly one-third of MEs in the service coming from a primary care background and the decoupling of the service from secondary care providers, both operationally and geographically, there is a strong basis for a straightforward non-acute roll out in the lead up to statutory implementation.

Overall, whilst facing the recognised challenges of implementation, the MES in Wales has been aided by the decision to adopt a single-service model for the whole nation with a single operational framework and digital system. The final phase of roll out is largely one of upscaling, in terms of numbers of cases reviewed and continued stakeholder engagement, to ensure that the service learns, adapts and improves as the implementation proceeds.

Example of an Acute Hospital Medical Examiner Service

The Norfolk and Norwich University Hospital (NNUH) is a 1200-bed teaching hospital providing care for a population of one million people. There are approximately 2500 deaths per annum. The NNUH established its MES in May 2019, initially staffed by MEs, until MEOs were recruited in June 2020.

Data show that around 97% of deaths were scrutinised in that time period. Figure 2.5 and Tables 2.1–2.3 show the workload and outcome of the NNUH MES from June 2020 to June 2021. This period covered a time when the coronavirus pandemic had commenced, and whilst MEOs were being trained and inducted for some time after their appointment. These data are used to provide an example of the nature and extent of the possible workload at a large acute hospital. The NNUH MES during this time had two whole-time equivalent MEOs and eight part-time MEs (a total of one whole-time equivalent), of whom one was Lead ME. The MEOs were from nursing and bereavement backgrounds, whilst the MEs were from a range of specialties, including general practice, vascular surgery, palliative care, and forensic and legal medicine. The NNUH MES works closely with, and is supported by, the bereavement service. The NNUH MES works closely with the

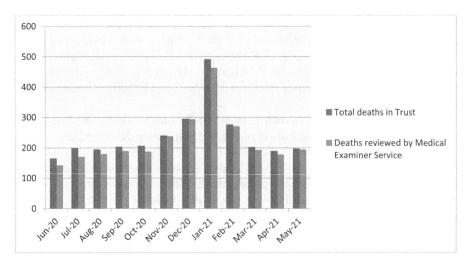

Figure 2.5 Summary of workload by month by the Medical Examiner Service at the Norfolk and Norwich University Hospitals NHS Trust from June 2020 to May 2021.[12]

Table 2.1 Summary of workload and outcome of cases scrutinised by the Medical Examiner Service at the Norfolk and Norwich University Hospitals NHS Trust from June 2020 to May 2021[12]

Workload of NNUH MES	1 June 2020 to 31 May 2021	% of deaths scrutinised (96.96% of total deaths)
Total number of deaths scrutinised	2775	
Non-HM Coroner cremations	1882	65.74
Non-HM Coroner burials	332	11.60
Other (Repatriation/body donation)	10	0.35
HM Coroner notifications	538	18.79
Form 100A issued by HM Coroner*	292	10.20
Post-mortem/Inquest	244	8.52
Paediatric deaths	11	0.38
Number of families who were spoken to	2394	83.62
Structured Judgement Review escalations	108	3.77
Patient Safety escalations	22	0.77

* Once a death is reported to HM Coroner, the Coroner must decide whether they have a duty to investigate the death, as set out in Section 1 Coroners and Justice Act 2009, and if it applies or not. The Coroner may decide, without a post-mortem, that the duty does not apply, and no further action is required. Form 100-A will be completed and sent to the registrar so that the registration of death process can be completed.

Table 2.2 Summary of notifications to HM Coroner by the Medical Examiner Service at the Norfolk and Norwich University Hospitals NHS Trust from June 2020 to May 2021[12]

	Number (data available - n=458)	%
Circumstance in which notification was made to HM Coroner under Regulation 3		
Use of medicinal product, controlled drug or psychoactive substance	3	0.66
Violence, trauma or injury	138	30.13
Self-harm/suicide	13	2.84
Neglect, including self-neglect	35	7.64
Treatment, procedure, surgery	103	22.49
Employment related	23	5.02
Unnatural	3	0.66
Cause of death unknown	132	28.82
Custody or state detention	8	1.75

Table 2.3 Summary of reasons for escalations to Structured Judgement Review by the Medical Examiner Service at the Norfolk and Norwich University Hospitals NHS Trust from June 2020 to May 2021[12]

	(n=108)	%
SJR escalations		
Significant family concerns	43	39.81
Staff/ME concerns	19	17.59
Learning disabilities/SMI	28	28.00
Elective	16	14.81
Homeless	2	1.85

local Mortality Governance System (MGS) and Learning from Deaths (LfD) framework. Pending the introduction of a national electronic software system, the NNUH ME-1B is integrated with, but independent of, the Mortality Governance System. Chapter 11 addresses the potential relationships between the MES, MGS and LfD. The roll out to the community will create a caseload of 6000 deaths per annum and will require a doubling of personnel.

Relationships with Other Teams Supporting the Deceased and Bereaved

The NME has been developing a Good Practice series focussing on specific aspects of the ME role. The first, 'How Medical Examiners can support people of Black, Asian and minority ethnic heritage and their relatives', provides recommendations that include: *'Medical Examiner should actively monitor trends and patterns for further action/health planning response, including whether outcomes for patients and relatives of those from Black, Asian and minority ethnic communities differ from those of other communities'*; and that *'Medical Examiners should be sensitive to the cultural and religious expectations and needs of all those who have suffered loss . . .'*.[13]

Good Practice Series Number 2 provides guidance on 'How Medical Examiners can facilitate urgent release of a body'. This advises on identifying which communities may have particular needs or wishes regarding timely release of a body and recommends working closely with other departments such as bereavement or the mortuary to undertake this. This may be used and adapted for those where death is anticipated and may be assisted by discussing the proposed cause of death in advance.[14]

Good Practice Series Number 3 provides guidance on 'Learning disability and autism' and the first two of seven recommendations are that MEs should *'Note the sensitivity of dealing with the death of someone who had a learning disability or who was autistic, and pay particular attention to support for carers who may for many years have been "the voice" and representative of the deceased'* and *'Remain conscious that a patient with a learning disability or who was autistic may have found it difficult to communicate with staff in hospitals and other health and care staff, and this may have had an impact on the cause of death and/or the events leading to death. Health inequalities arising from a person having a learning disability or who was autistic may have contributed to the death.'*[15]

Good Practice Series Number 4 covers organ and tissue donation, encouraging MES to establish links with organ donation teams to minimise delays, while ensuring that full ME scrutiny takes place.[16]

Good Practice Series Number 5 provides guidance on post-mortem examinations, including understanding the different types of examination, their benefits and limitations, and when each is appropriate. *It is not part of the role of medical examiners to commission or conduct post-mortem examinations, and they should not encroach on coroners' judicial prerogative to determine when they think a post-mortem examination is required. However, the medical examiner system may impact further by reducing the number of unnecessary post-mortem examinations [. . .] by increasing the appropriateness of referrals made to coroners.*[17]

Good Practice Series Number 6 is on the topic of medical examiners and child deaths. There was particularly wide stakeholder engagement and consultation on this document, which focuses on how MEs interact with the existing statutory child death investigation processes. *Medical examiners are not a replacement for other processes and should neither complicate matters nor generate unnecessary bureaucracy.*[18]

Good Practice Series Number 7 looks at mental health and eating disorders, highlighting the role that MEs can play in identifying links between causes of death and mental health conditions, particularly ensuring that MCCDs are completing accurately and identifying opportunities for learning to improve future care.[19]

Good Practice Series Number 8 explores the role of MEs in antimicrobial resistance, particularly in improving the accuracy of death certification.[16]

These guidance documents are very helpful in addressing questions and matters of concern that arise on a frequent basis within the ME setting.

Conclusions

The ME system represents a new process in the medicolegal investigation of death in England and Wales. Its threefold main aims – to provide bereaved families with greater transparency and opportunities to raise concerns; to improve the quality/accuracy of medical certification of cause of death; and to ensure referrals to coroners are appropriate –appear to be being achieved. The national roll out of a new system in April 2019 could have been thwarted by the coronavirus pandemic, but far from being thwarted, appears to have given added impetus. Training and recruitment of MEs and MEOs, and the establishment of local ME services working closely with bereavement, mortuary, coronial and registration services has been achieved within a two-year period. Although far from complete, progress has been rapid, and the next phase of community death scrutiny will begin to achieve the aim of all non-coronial deaths being reviewed by independent MEs, supported by trained MEOs.

REFERENCES

1. National Medical Examiner. Implementing the Medical Examiner System: National Medical Examiner's good practice guidelines, 2020. https://www.england.nhs.uk/wp-content/uploads/2020/08/National_Medical_Examiner_-_good_practice_guidelines.pdf (accessed 17 December 2021).

2. NHS England & NHS Improvement. System Letter: Extending medical examiner scrutiny to non-acute settings, 2021. https://www.england.nhs.uk/wp-content/uploads/2021/06/B0477-extending-medical-examiner-scrutiny-to-non-acute-settings.pdf (accessed 17 December 2021).

3. Health and Care Act 2022. www.legislation.gov.uk/ukpga/2022/31/contents/enacted (accessed 13 June 2022)

4. Ministry of Justice. Notification of Deaths Regulations 2019 Guidance, 2019. https://www.gov.uk/government/publications/notification-of-deaths-regulations-2019-guidance (accessed 17 December 2021).

5. Royal College of Pathologists. Cause of Death List, 2020. https://www.rcpath.org/uploads/assets/c16ae453-6c63-47ff-8c45fd2c56521ab9/G199-Cause-of-death-list.pdf (accessed 17 December 2021).

6. Office of National Statistics. Guidance for Doctors Completing Medical Certificates of Cause of Death in England and Wales, 2020. https://assets.publishing.service.gov.uk/government/uploads/system/uploads/attachment_data/file/877302/guidance-for-doctors-completing-medical-certificates-of-cause-of-death-covid-19.pdf (accessed 17 December 2021).

7. GOV.uk. Coroners and Justice Act, 2009. https://www.legislation.gov.uk/ukpga/2009/25/data.pdf (accessed 17 December 2021).

8. GOV.uk. Coronavirus Act, 2020. https://www.legislation.gov.uk/ukpga/2020/7/contents/enacted (accessed 17 December 2021).

9. NHS England & NHS Improvement. Coronavirus Act – excess death provisions: information and guidance for medical practitioners, 2020. https://www.england.nhs.uk/coronavirus/wp-content/uploads/sites/52/2020/03/COVID-19-Act-excess-death-provisions-info-and-guidance-31-03-20.pdf (accessed 17 December 2021).

10. Francis R. Report of the Mid-Staffordshire NHS Foundation Trust Public Inquiry, 2013. https://www.gov.uk/government/publications/report-of-the-mid-staffordshire-nhs-foundation-trust-public-inquiry (accessed 17 December 2021).

11. Palmer S. Review of the Use of Risk Adjusted Mortality Data in NHS Wales, 2014. https://gov.wales/written-statement-publication-professor-stephen-palmers-review-use-risk-adjusted-mortality-data-nhs (accessed 13 July 2022).

12. Payne-James JJ, Parapanos L, Carpenter K, Lopez B. The workload of a medical examiner service at an acute National Health Service hospital during the COVID-19 pandemic: The Norfolk & Norwich University Hospital experience. Medicine, Science & the Law, March 2022 https://doi.org/10.1177/00258024221087005

13. National Medical Examiner. National Medical Examiner's Good Practice Series No. 1. How medical examiners can support people of Black, Asian and minority ethnic heritage and their relatives, 2021. https://www.rcpath.org/uploads/assets/72675084-5ed3-43a1-b518c61395dd1194/Good-Practice-Series-BAME-paper.pdf (accessed 17 December 2021).

14. National Medical Examiner. National Medical Examiner's Good Practice Series No. 2. How medical examiners can facilitate urgent release of a body, 2021. https://www.rcpath.org/uploads/assets/3590bf7f-a43e-4248-980640c5c12354c4/Good-Practice-Series-Urgent-release-of-a-bodyFor-Publication.pdf (accessed 17 December 2021).

15. National Medical Examiner. National Medical Examiner's Good Practice Series No. 3. Learning disability and autism, 2021. https://www.rcpath.org/uploads/assets/daf86eaa-d591-40d5-99d54118d10444d2/Good-Practice-Series-Learning-disability-and-autism-For-Publication.pdf (accessed 17 December 2021).

16. National Medical Examiner. National Medical Examiner's Good Practice Series No. 4. Organ and tissue donation. October 2021 https://www.rcpath.org/uploads/assets/12d79507-48e1-4ae7-858615f0327da5c1/Good-Practice-Series-Organ-and-tissue-donation.pdf (accessed 20 June 2022).

17. National Medical Examiner. National Medical Examiner's Good Practice Series No. 5. Post-mortem examinations. March 2022 https://www.rcpath.org/uploads/assets/6f3bffc0-f30b-4053-8d50fb2b5df0e57c/Good-Practice-Series-Post-mortem-examinationsFor-Publication.pdf (accessed 20 June 2022).
18. National Medical Examiner. National Medical Examiner's Good Practice Series No. 6. Medical examiners and child deaths. March 2022 https://www.rcpath.org/uploads/assets/7fa7a9d6-ada5-4597-b16f4602c93d3e91/Good-Practice-Series-Child-Deaths.pdf (accessed 20 June 2022).
19. National Medical Examiner. National Medical Examiner's Good Practice Series No.7. Mental Health and Eating Disorders. July 2022 https://www.rcpath.org/profession/medical-examiners/good-practice-series.html

CHAPTER 3

The Role of the Regional Medical Examiner and Regional Medical Examiner Officer

Ellen Makings and Siobhan Costello

Structure of National and Regional Medical Examiner Team

Dr Alan Fletcher, the National Medical Examiner for England and Wales, was appointed in March 2019. The National Medical Examiner Office was established and over the course of that year, Regional Medical Examiners and Regional Medical Examiner Officers were appointed to regional posts in England and Wales.

England is divided into seven NHS regions (Figure 3.1) . Each region has a Regional Medical Examiner and a Regional Medical Examiner Officer. These roles are part-time and 0.4 full-time equivalent (15 hours a week). Table 3.1 shows the number of acute Trusts in each of these regions.

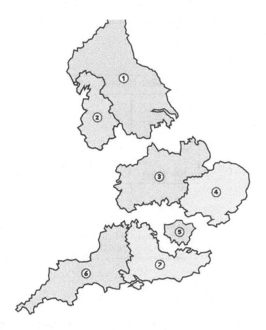

Figure 3.1   Seven NHS regions in England. 1. North East and Yorkshire; 2. North West; 3. Midlands; 4. East of England; . London; 6. South West; 7. South East.

DOI: 10.1201/9781003188759-3

Table 3.1 Number of acute trusts in each region (England)

Region	Number of acute trusts
North East and Yorkshire	22
North West	20
Midlands	42
East	17
London	39
South East	20
South West	16

Regional Medical Examiners are senior registered medical practitioners (doctors) who have experience in leadership roles and have worked with or have been part of a Medical Examiner office.

The National and Regional Medical Examiner teams are employed by NHS England. The Regional Medical Examiner is accountable to the National Medical Examiner and is responsible for overseeing the implementation and provision of Medical Examiner offices in their region. Figure 3.2 shows the infrastructure for the National Medical Examiner Service.

The Regional Medical Examiner team works closely with the National Medical Examiner, providing them with updates of progress of local trust Medical Examiner offices. Regular meetings take place between the regional teams and the National Medical Examiner team to discuss next steps in the development

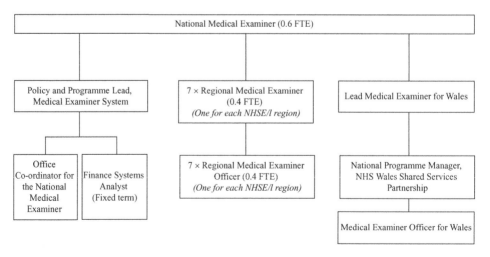

Figure 3.2 Infrastructure for the National Medical Examiner Service. From *Implementing the Medical Examiner System: National Medical Examiner's good practice guidelines*. NHSI. January 2020.[2]

of the service and share information regarding national policy and development of the Medical Examiner service nationally. These meetings are also an opportunity for other members of the national team to give a regional update and share examples of good practice or help solve problems encountered at a regional level.

Routes of Escalation

The Regional Medical Examiner provides an independent line of advice and accountability for Medical Examiners working in their region.

A Medical Examiner may raise a concern if they are not satisfied by the response to that concern when it is raised within the employing NHS trust, or if the Medical Examiner feels that their independent role is being challenged or compromised.

The Regional Medical Examiner has various options to address such concerns when they are raised and will choose the most appropriate. Often the NHS trust Medical Director is contacted and a successful solution may be reached with collaborative working. If a solution is not achieved, the Regional Medical Examiner will then seek support from the NHS Regional Medical Director and in some cases, directly from the National Medical Examiner.

The Role of the Regional Medical Examiner

A key role of the Regional Medical Examiner is overseeing the provision and development of the multiple Medical Examiner services within their region.

All 129 acute trusts in England now have an ME service. Implementation has progressed at different rates in different trusts, and to some extent these services have developed from the ground up rather than the top down, but since May 2019 they have done so with broad guidance from the National Medical Examiner. The Medical Examiner service was first proposed by Dame Janet Smith DBE in 2005 in her report The Shipman Inquiry, Third Report: Death certification and the investigation of deaths by Coroners[1] following the Shipman enquiry (see also Chapter 1). Seven pilot sites were established to test out the new proposals. The pilot schemes ranged from small initiatives in specific communities (e.g. Inner North London, Powys, Leicester) to large programmes covering primary and secondary care, adult, perinatal and neonatal deaths (e.g. Sheffield). The smaller pilots lasted several months, the larger ones continued for over a decade and merged with early implementation of the current scheme. These were in Sheffield, Gloucester, Powys, Inner North London, Leicester, Brighton & Hove and Mid_ Essex. A report of the outcome of the pilot schemes was published by the Royal College of Pathologists in 2016.[3] Several of these pilot sites continued to provide their services after the pilot had ceased and neighbouring hospitals soon learned of the benefits the trusts were seeing from running such a service in the non-statutory setting, so further Medical Examiner offices were established.

The Regional Medical Examiner teams have worked closely with all of the acute hospital providers to assist with the formation of their own local Medical Examiner offices. This has involved a variety of support including job descriptions, assistance with interviews, use of documentation for scrutinies, finance modelling and the actual process of carrying out the three parts of the process:

1. Independent scrutiny of the notes
2. Discussion with the doctor agreeing causes of death
3. Discussion with relatives about the proposed causes of death and any concerns or questions they have.

The Regional Medical Examiner team will often assist in the interview process for the appointment of Medical Examiners and Medical Examiner Officers. This is particularly helpful if the office is newly opened and there may be a lack of knowledge or expertise surrounding the Medical Examiner system.

Having established the Medical Examiner offices, the next step, which is currently in process, is to support the development of the scrutiny of those deaths outside the acute hospital setting in the community (for example at home, in nursing homes and in community hospitals). The Regional Medical Examiner team plays a vital role in this development as support will be required to undertake a major change in the death notification process, which has been in place for many years. It is key that the independence of the Medical Examiner role is highlighted in the engagement process and that although acute NHS trusts host the office, the Medical Examiner service has its own governance structure with accountability for scrutiny of community deaths externally to the National Medical Examiner via the Regional Medical Examiner, in the same way as for acute NHS trust deaths.

The Role of the Regional Medical Examiner Officer

The role of the Regional Medical Examiner Officer is to support the Regional Medical Examiner to establish and maintain a high-quality Medical Examiner service, both within acute trusts and across the community of a given region.

The Regional Medical Examiner Officer, together with the Regional Medical Examiner, is accountable for the establishment of each Medical Examiner service through strategic and operational planning and programme management. This management will ensure that each Medical Examiner Service is maintained effectively, taking into account geography and demographics, ensuring an equitable service so that all of the region has access to a Medical Examiner Service.

Regional Medical Examiner Officers facilitate discussions with stakeholders across acute and community settings such as faith groups, patient and family representatives and other regional stakeholders. At these discussions, complex and sensitive arrangements can be negotiated and agreed between organisations in relation to the provision of the Medical Examiner service or around the quality of care provided to deceased patients.

Regional Medical Examiners also liaise with senior Coroners, Coroner's officers and registration services to ensure effective communication and smooth processes exist between them and Medical Examiner Services.

The Regional Medical Examiner Officer supports Medical Examiner offices in the recruitment of Medical Examiner Officers by giving advice on organisational structure, pay scales and management. The Regional Medical Examiner Officer can advise and participate in the shortlisting and interviewing of potential candidates. The Regional Medical Examiner Officer provides ongoing support to Medical Examiner Officers in post across the region through the provision of regular fora so that Medical Examiner Officers across the region can network, engage with and support each other. The Regional Medical Examiner Officer will also arrange induction meetings with new Medical Examiner Officers to introduce them to the region and inform them of current national and regional issues. The Regional Medical Examiner Officer will also act as a source of contact to other Medical Examiner Officers and stakeholders across the region and will provide expert advice on the Medical Examiner system.

The Regional Medical Examiner Officer assists the National Programme Lead in the development of information materials for the Medical Examiner service. This includes information for the establishment of the service within the acute and community settings. The Regional Medical Examiner Officer is responsible for organising meetings to bring together Medical Examiners and Medical Examiner Officers from all NHS trusts across their region, such as online or face-to-face fora to discuss key issues and provide support, networking and training. The fact that these functions are able to be undertaken remotely allowed the Medical Examiner system to continue to function and develop throughout the COVID-19 pandemic. The Regional Medical Examiner Officers supports all Medical Examiner services across the region in producing accurate quarterly reporting of activity and advising on the establishment of the Medical Examiner IT systems.

Together, the Regional Medical Examiner and the Regional Medical Examiner Officers act as a direct reporting line to the National Medical Examiner on matters such as trends and clinical governance, and brief the National Medical Examiner on issues of concern or on successes of local Medical Examiner Services.

Skills of the Regional Medical Examiner Officer

The Regional Medical Examiner Officer requires extensive experience in working at a senior level in the NHS or a related organisation. Regional Medical Examiner Officers may come from a clinical background such as nursing or might have a risk management, clinical governance or legal background, or have held a lead role in dealing with complaints or patient experience within an NHS trust.

Regional Medical Examiner Officers must have experience of working across systems at a regional level and of managing complex programmes of work, be skilled in working with and influencing stakeholders, and providing advice and guidance to people for whom they do not have direct line management responsibilities.

Key Relationships at Regional Level

The Medical Examiner system presents a significant change to the bereavement process paperwork and so it is important that all external key stakeholders are identified so that Regional Medical Examiner teams can build relationships and share information to explain the role and the impact it is likely to have on other parts of the service.

HM Coroner service

The Regional Medical Examiner can play an important role in developing good working relationships with the Coroner and Coroner's office. They can facilitate meetings with the Coroner and the Medical Examiner offices within their jurisdiction, to provide an opportunity to discuss ways of working and how they would like to communicate with each other. This will differ in areas as various methods are used for Coroner's referrals currently.

The Regional Medical Examiner Officer can also work with Coroner's officers to explain the role of the Medical Examiner Officer and how they can support each other.

Registration services

Liaising with registration services in the region will provide registrars with a good understanding of the Medical Examiner role. Concerns have been raised that the Medical Examiner service will have a negative impact on the timeline given for registration of death. It is important to explain that the system has a number of expected benefits. These include: improved accuracy of the Medical Certificate of Cause of Death (MCCD); fewer MCCD rejections requiring referral to the Coroner; and providing better information and explanations to bereaved families so that they can understand the causes of death, as these will have been explained by the Medical Examiner Service.

Locally agreed initiatives may develop whilst in the non-statutory phase such as the Medical Examiner initialling and dating the MCCD to indicate that the medical records have been scrutinised, and that the causes of death have been discussed and agreed with the doctor completing the MCCD.

Coronavirus

The coronavirus pandemic had a large impact on bereavement services from March 2020 onwards. This was a time when many Medical Examiner offices had become established and were gradually getting to grips with the new process. This caused the Medical Examiner offices in acute NHS trusts to take on slightly different roles linked to the easements in the death process as documented in the Coronavirus Act 2020.[4]

The rapid changes in the death registration process led to Regional Medical Examiner teams working closely with their offices across the region. The use of online collaboration tools such as MS Teams and Zoom enabled regular virtual meetings to take place between Regional Medical Examiner teams and local Medical Examiner services throughout the pandemic, to provide updates regarding changes in the process and pastoral support during what was a particularly stressful time for bereavement services, which were dealing with a far larger workload than in normal practice. It also laid the foundations for a robust, supportive network and a place to share learning and good practice, and was welcomed by local Medical Examiner Services. ME services have also been well placed to support colleagues through the legislative changes at the end of the Coronavirus Act 2020, with a return to previous guidance with the exception of several pandemic easements which have been retained permanently.

The NHS England and NHS Improvement website provides contact details for national and regional teams.[5]

The Future

As Medical Examiner offices mature and become established with a good period of stability in workload, the role of the Regional Medical Examiner team will evolve. The regional teams will continue to provide clinical support, recruitment advice and other functions as previously, but the focus will change to one of ensuring quality assurance of the Medical Examiner processes supported by robust clinical governance frameworks to deal with any concerns raised around hospital and community deaths.

REFERENCES

1. Dame Janet Smith. The Shipman Inquiry, Third Report: Death certification and the investigation of deaths by Coroners, 2003. https://www.gov.uk/government/uploads/system/uploads/attachment_data/file/273227/5854.pdf (accessed 17 December 2021).
2. NHS. Implementing the Medical Examiner System: National Medical Examiner's good practice guidelines, 2020. https://www.england.nhs.uk/wp-content/uploads/2020/08/National_Medical_Examiner_-_good_practice_guidelines.pdf (accessed 17 December 2021).

3. Department of Health. Reforming Death Certification: Introducing scrutiny by Medical Examiners: Lessons from the pilots of the reforms set out in the Coroners and Justice Act, *2009*, 2016. https://assets.publishing.service.gov.uk/government/uploads/system/uploads/attachment_data/file/521226/Death_certificate_reforms_pilots_-_report_A.pdf?msclkid=7c68c6d3af551 1ecad1afc4b1d2c2cad (accessed 17 December 2021).

4. GOV.uk. Coronavirus Act, 2020. https://www.legislation.gov.uk/ukpga/2020/7/contents/enacted (accessed 17 December 2021).

5. NHS England and NHS Improvement. The National Medical Examiner System, 2021. https://www.england.nhs.uk/establishing-medical-examiner-system-nhs/#national-and-regional-contacts (accessed 17 December 2021).

CHAPTER 4

The Role of the Medical Examiner

Golda Shelley-Fraser

Introduction

The principal role of a Medical Examiner (ME) is to scrutinise non-coronial deaths during the immediate few days after death has occurred. The process of independent ME scrutiny seeks to establish the cause of death, determine whether the death needs to be notified to a Coroner and direct any care concerns raised. This process ensures compliance with the procedural and legal requirements for death registration and investigation by Coroners where necessary.

ME scrutiny has three components: review of the deceased's medical records by a Medical Examiner; communication with the certifying doctor; and discussion with the next of kin or informant.

Medical Examiner Scrutiny

Review of the medical record

Scrutiny of the medical record is a fact-finding, information-gathering exercise. This component of the scrutiny process should ideally be performed first. It entails a proportionate review of the medical record and should be a thorough, methodical and targeted process, focused on the final hospital admission or most recent episodes of care.

Most importantly, when starting the review, the ME must always ensure that they have the correct patient's medical record. Then begin with the basics: name of the deceased, date of birth, date and time of death, and address. With just these few pieces of data, the ME can begin processing the information.

The age of the deceased gives an indication of the likelihood of certain disease processes. The address, whether a private residence or care home, may provide information regarding performance status. Also, an ME may be aware of known concerns about particular care homes or other facilities.

Other core data items to note when scrutinising the medical record are what symptoms or condition brought the patient into a care setting, any comorbidities, and

DOI: 10.1201/9781003188759-4

the past medical history, drug history and occupation, which can provide useful information on the likelihood of industrial disease.

In addition to the medical notes, radiology and pathology reports and blood results can all provide valuable information. For in-patient deaths, the nursing records can provide essential information about in-patient falls, pressure sores and a range of safeguarding issues. Drug charts and fluid balance charts may also be of relevance.

Throughout the entire review process, the ME must stay alert to identify any factors which may indicate an unnatural death. On reviewing the clinical record, any documented concerns raised by the team providing care or family members should be noted.

This review process will provide the ME with a summary of the deceased's pre-morbid state, the events leading up to the death, the nature of the death and whether it was expected or sudden.

The time needed to complete this review will very much depend on the volume of information available and the complexity of the case. It could vary from as little as 10 minutes to beyond an hour, dependent on the nature of the case and any care issues that arise. The format of information available to the ME will also vary depending on whether the death occurred in an acute hospital setting, a non-acute care-providing organisation or at home.

The medical record may take the form of a physical set of notes, an electronic patient record or a combination of the two. These may be brief (for example, a death taking place in an emergency department) or voluminous (for example, a death of an elderly patient with multiple comorbidities and a prolonged in-hospital stay). Irrespective of where the death has occurred or the type of patient record available, the attention to detail and quality of scrutiny should be of the same high standard.

By the end of this component of the scrutiny process, the ME should ideally have a clear understanding of the cause of death, whether there is a requirement for notification to the Coroner and if there are any concerns that need to be raised.

Communication with the qualified attending practitioner/certifying doctor

The purpose of this component of the ME scrutiny process is to agree the cause of death with the certifying doctor and ensure the accuracy of the Medical Certificate of Cause of Death (MCCD). Communication with the designated care-providing doctor may take a variety of forms, including a face-to-face discussion in the ME office, a phone call or an email. For those straightforward cases where the cause of death is clear, it is perfectly acceptable for the certifying doctor to provide a proposed cause of death via email or over the phone to a Medical Examiner Officer

(MEO), negating the need for a conversation with the ME, if agreed upon. The latter is likely to be the most common interaction for uncomplicated deaths that occur within the non-acute sector.

Within acute NHS trusts, the certifying doctor, also termed the qualified attending practitioner (QAP) (terms that are used interchangeably throughout this book), is often a non-consultant grade, and acts as representative of the clinical care providing team. It is of benefit to the process if the clinical team (including the consultant) have had a discussion regarding the proposed cause of death in advance of the QAP speaking to the ME.

Communication with the QAP is of most value to the ME when it follows the ME scrutiny of the medical record, to reduce the possibly of bias. This also gives the ME the opportunity to ask questions relating to any queries that have arisen whilst scrutinising the clinical notes. It is also essential to ask the certifying doctor if they have any concerns at all about the care provided to the deceased during their final admission or most recent care episode.

During this interaction, the QAP will ideally present their proposed cause of death. If agreed upon, this component of the scrutiny process is complete. However, occasionally, a QAP may be unable to offer a proposed cause of death. This may arise if the case is particularly complex or if there are uncertainties related to the cause of death. One of the roles of the ME is to support certifying doctors with the terminology and order of pathologies on the MCCD, but it is not the ME's role to instruct certifying doctors what to write.[1] If the QAP has some gaps in their knowledge about the case that prevent them from proposing a cause of death, they should revise the case notes and if necessary, speak with their senior clinical team members for support and advice. They complete the MCCD to the 'best of their knowledge and belief', not to the best of the Medical Examiner's knowledge and belief.

It may be that a certifying doctor contacts the ME before there has been the opportunity for the ME to scrutinise the clinical notes. This may be for advice regarding the cause of death or whether a death needs to be notified to a Coroner. This is acceptable and sometimes unavoidable when the QAP may not be available later due to shift patterns or leave. However, in these instances, the ME must remain alert to the fact that the certifying doctor's account may be limited to their knowledge and perspective of the case and may not provide a thorough unbiased account of the death. In these circumstances, it is important for the ME to lead the conversation and ask a series of standardised questions to get a balanced overview of the case. It is also important to not let this upfront communication with the QAP influence the subsequent scrutiny of the medical record.

One of the key roles of MEs is to ensure the accuracy of the MCCD and contribute to the education and training of certifying doctors in the understanding of death certification. MEs should be prepared and offer to teach and speak at educational events to contribute to wider learning and understanding of death certification as part of patient care.

Discussion with the bereaved/informant

The ME system aims to put the bereaved at the heart of the process. It does this by ensuring that the cause of death is explained and discussed openly and the bereaved are given an opportunity to ask questions and raise any concerns they may have had relating to the care of the deceased. This is the final component of the scrutiny process and for many MEs and MEOs is (perhaps surprisingly to many observers) the most rewarding and valuable aspect of the role.

This conversation with the bereaved generally takes place by phone, which can bring with it some challenges. The bereaved or informant (the term used for the person who registers the death) is likely to have been told already by the ME office or bereavement team to expect a phone call from an ME. An ME should prepare for the conversation by ensuring that that have the contact details for the correct person and that they are in a quiet space away from background noise. At the start of the call, the ME should introduce themself and establish whether it is an acceptable time to have the discussion. MEs should offer condolences at the beginning of the conversation and explain that their ME role is as an independent doctor who was not part of the treating team, and that they were not known to the deceased.

When talking through the cause of death, it is important to read out the proposed cause of death and offer to explain the medical terminology if wanted. The ME should establish whether the wording is in keeping with what the bereaved or informant was expecting and in line what the care providing team had told them.

If the bereaved is not content with the proposed cause of death, the ME should try to establish why. Is there a particular word or term they object to? It may simply be that a clinical team used lay terms to try and explain what had happened to their loved one, which may differ substantially from the medical terminology. Do they feel that a significant pathology or disease process or condition or event has not been properly represented? Whilst the role of the ME is to ensure the overall accuracy of the MCCD, it may be that a change in terminology, however minor, makes all the difference to the bereaved. For instance, 'alcohol-related liver disease' may be more acceptable than 'alcoholic liver disease' and makes little difference from an accuracy perspective. The ME should listen to their concerns and explain sensitively the importance of transparency and accuracy of the wording on the MCCD.

The ME then ascertains whether the bereaved or informant has any questions or concerns about the care the deceased received before death. When questions relate to the specific details of the care, it is often preferable for these to be addressed by the care-providing team rather than the ME and so advice on how to arrange such a meeting is most useful. Any concerns raised by the bereaved or informant should be documented and addresed as appropriate. Verbatim quotes are very helpful. Frequently, the bereaved give positive feedback about the care provided by individuals and teams and it is important to ensure that is passed on too.

It is important for the ME to anticipate that these conversations can sometimes be difficult. The ME should refer to the scrutiny of the medical record and make a note of names of family members who raised concerns at the time, as they may be the next of kin the ME will be speaking to. The bereaved may be upset or angry and in a state of shock. MEs need to be empathic, listen attentively and consider offering to call back later if necessary. If an ME has any concerns about the bereaved they speak to, perhaps if they have an exaggerated grief reaction or are in a fragile emotional state, the ME should inform a member of the bereavement team, who are skilled and will be able to provide the bereaved with the necessary support.

It is important for an ME to develop their own style for these conversations and to be authentic. It can be extremely useful to listen to ME and MEO colleagues during such conversations and likewise seek feedback from members of the ME team.

The ME is accountable for all three components of the scrutiny process, but it is acceptable to delegate two of the three components of ME scrutiny to an MEO. Communication with the medical team and discussion with the bereaved can be performed by an MEO under the authority of the ME; however, the medical record scrutiny component must be performed by the ME.[1]

Referral to the Coroner

MEs should establish strong working relationships with their local Coroner and Coroner's officers.

The Notification of Deaths Regulations 2019[2] sets out the types of death that should be referred to a Coroner. Many deaths requiring notification to a Coroner may bypass the Medical Examiner Service (MES). Some Coroners request that all definite and possible coronial notifications must be reviewed by the local MES.

However, a proportion of deaths that undergo ME scrutiny will require notification to the Coroner. Such cases may include sudden and unexpected natural deaths where the cause of death is uncertain or not known, and deaths that occurred following a surgical procedure or an unnatural event such as a fall.

When scrutinising a case, the ME should always be alert to information and/or circumstances that may warrant a notification (referral) to a Coroner.[3] It is important to note the occupation of the deceased when considering certain pathologies that may be attributable to their employment, such as asbestos-related lung disease. If this is not in the medical records, it may be something to be asked in discussion with the family. Other examples include conditions where a natural pathology is attributable to a previous unnatural event, such as a case of bronchopneumonia in a patient who was paralysed because of trauma many decades previously or a seizure-related death secondary to traumatic brain injury from an assault.

If a cause of death is known and natural but there is an unnatural event that is considered to be contributory in the death within Part 2 of the MCCD, the case would require referral to the Coroner, who is likely to issue a Form 100A. Such cases will undergo the full ME scrutiny process in addition to being notified to the Coroner. An example of such a case would be:

1a. Haemorrhagic stroke
1b. Hypertension
2. High international normalised ratio on warfarin for atrial fibrillation.

Where the effects of anticoagulation have contributed to the haemorrhagic stroke, a Coroner's notification is necessary. The Coroner may issue a Form 100A, allowing the QAP to issue the medical certificate without a post-mortem examination or inquest.

Occasionally cases are complex and nuanced and, even for an experienced ME, it may not be clear whether a case should be referred to a Coroner or not. A good working relationship with the Coroner's office, with clear and agreed methods of communication, will prove invaluable in these instances. For some MESs, a quick phone call to the Coroner may allow a brief discussion of the case and a recommendation about whether a case should be formally referred or not. Senior Coroners may vary in their interpretation of the notification guidelines, although there is less variation than previously.

Coroners will benefit from the ME system in that the quality and appropriateness of referrals should improve. Parenthetically, with increased consistency and accuracy of MCCDs, there should be fewer MCCDs rejected by registration services, which would have otherwise been notified to a Coroner.

It is anticipated that the ME will be used by referring clinicians and Coroners as a medical advice resource and many Coroners are already doing this.

Raising Concerns

One of the aims of the ME scrutiny process is to highlight any concerns raised and escalate them appropriately using an agreed and consistent method.[1]

When scrutinising a death, MEs should stay alert to concerns, which should be passed via NHS clinical governance streams. Does the medical record document any issues that are a cause for concern? Has the certifying doctor raised any concerns? Have the bereaved voiced any concerns about the care their loved one received prior to death?

The nature of concerns an ME will come across will vary from minor (those that did not affect clinical outcome, although they are of concern to either the family or the certifying doctor) to the more serious. Minor concerns may include frequent bed transfers of patients, poor communication between clinical staff, inability of family or carers to contact wards, inability of family or carers to speak to a doctor and omissions to non-essential medications. More serious concerns may include failure to provide basic care, evidence of neglect and significant complications following an elective procedure where the outcome was, or may have been, affected.

When a patient dies in an acute NHS trust setting, in line with Learning from Deaths,[4] there are specific criteria that warrant referring a case for a structured judgement review (SJR), for example deaths of those with learning disabilities, deaths following an elective procedure, and maternal and neonatal deaths, in addition to those where concerns have been raised and noted during the scrutiny process. Some of these cases may also require notification to a Coroner. Individual care-providing organisations may have their own additional criteria for review due to local patient safety initiatives, and the MES should be aware of and follow these.

Monitoring and investigation are not part of the MES role and the MES may not necessarily receive any feedback on referrals into clinical governance streams, although it should be encouraged. If there are concerns or trends regarding an organisation, these should be escalated to the Regional Medical Examiner, or the Lead Medical Examiner for Wales, for consideration and investigation.[1]

Registrars of Births and Deaths

One other aim of the ME system is to improve the quality, accuracy and consistency of the MCCD.[1] The Cause of Death List[5] details many of the common conditions that may, or may not, be included on the MCCD without coronial referral. This is not an exhaustive list of all possible causes of death, but includes many of the causes that have caused confusion in the past.

When supporting the certifying doctor in writing the MCCD, it is important that the cause of death is structured appropriately on the MCCD in accordance with the World Health Organisation (WHO) recommendations (I(a), I(b), I(c) and part II)[6] and that the correct (acceptable) terminology is used. This is to ensure that the MCCD is not rejected by the registration office and subsequently referred to the Coroner. A rejected MCCD can be upsetting for the bereaved or informant, resulting in distress and delays to registration and funeral arrangements.

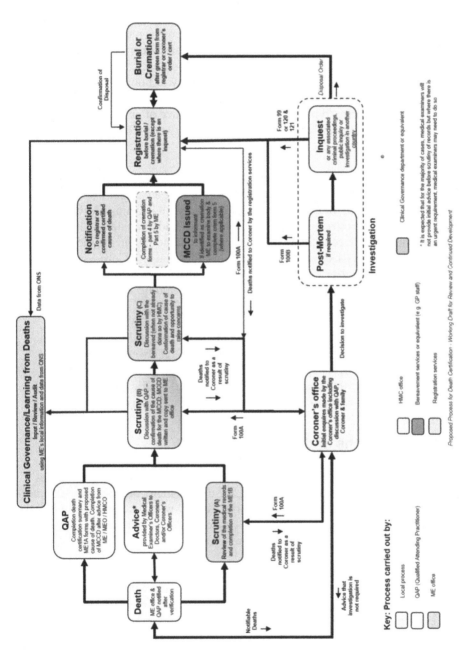

Figure 4.1 Overview of proposed process for death certification.

It is essential, as with other key stakeholders, to establish good working relationships and communication with the local registration service. Any rejected MCCDs should be fed back to the ME office and the individual ME to be used as a learning point and reflected on.

Independence

Independence is key to the ME role and function. MEs are senior registered medical practitioners of at least five years' standing and in most cases are hospital consultants or general practitioners. They are employed by the host acute NHS trust in which the ME office is located but funded by NHS England.[1]

The duty of an ME is to act independently of the host trust, for the deceased and bereaved, and to ensure that if required, a referral to the Coroner is made, that the MCCD is accurate and that any clinical governance concerns are raised.

The ME must ensure that they are not biased in any way when scrutinising a death. Any conflict or perceived potential conflict of interest should be avoided. For these reasons, it is not appropriate to scrutinise a death when the ME, their clinical team or department has been involved in the treatment of the deceased in any capacity. Likewise, if an ME has a close professional or any personal relationship with a colleague who has been involved in the deceased's care it is appropriate that the case is dealt with by another ME. In a similar vein, those MEs who are also practising post-mortem pathologists should not perform a post-mortem on a case where they were involved in the Coroner's referral.[1]

MEs must not have had prior conversations with the bereaved about the deceased in a clinical capacity prior to the death. When speaking to the bereaved, the ME should state that they are an independent doctor, to provide reassurance and facilitate open and transparent conversation regarding any concerns.

It is not appropriate for an ME to also be a mortality lead within an NHS trust as there may be a conflict of interest with respect to clinical governance referrals.[1] If in their clinical role an ME performs SJRs, it is not good practice to review a case on which they performed ME scrutiny.

Ultimately, the ME and others should be comfortable that there is no conflict of interest or potential bias through relationship with a patient, a colleague or the bereaved when scrutinising a case.

Prioritisation of Cases

MEs should work as effectively and efficiently as possible and prioritise their case load as necessary. The General Register Office (GRO) requires by law that deaths are registered within five calendar days (not working days) unless the death is referred to the Coroner. ME scrutiny should not cause any unnecessary delays to the death registration process or cause any additional anxiety to the bereaved or informant.[1] ME scrutiny should also not cause unnecessary delays when referring to a Coroner. Establishing ways of working to communicate with the QAP and the bereaved in a timely fashion is important.

Some deaths may require urgent release of the body and the MES should be able to facilitate this by provide an evening and weekend out-of-hours service. Establishing links with faith communities, paediatric services and organ donation services, and setting up protocols to fit local needs for urgent release cases, is recommended.[1]

Whilst serving the population and the requirements for urgent release of bodies, it is important for MEs to maintain attention to detail and integrity of the scrutiny process in all cases without compromise on quality.

Documentation

All aspects of ME scrutiny should be recorded accurately, either using the exemplar forms available, ME-1 (Part1)[7] and ME-1 (Part B),[8] or an alternative local version. Whether in paper or electronic form, the information should be stored securely and should not form part of the deceased's clinical record.

ME scrutiny should be recorded with the knowledge that it may be subject to auditing processes and may be viewed by other parties for the purposes of clinical governance reviews and/or Coroner's investigations. It may also be discoverable in litigation.

ME offices also have a duty to record information that is required by the National Medical Examiner team for quarterly and annual reporting exercises.[1]

A digital ME system for England is currently in development. In the future it is intended that all MEs and MEOs in England will have access to this, with the expectation that all ME scrutiny will be recorded on the national digital system.

Coronavirus Act 2020

The Coronavirus Act 2020 introduced easements to death certification processes and cremation forms as part of the emergency provisions during the COVID-19 pandemic.[9] It expired at midnight on 24 March 2022.[10]

Undoubtedly, the easements impacted and shaped many aspects of the ME scrutiny process. Helpfully for the ME system, following expiration of the Act, some of the changes have been retained on a permanent basis.

The period of time before death within which a doctor completing a Medical Certificate of Cause of Death (MCCD) must have seen a deceased patient remains at 28 days. Prior to the coronavirus pandemic, the limit was 14 days. It remains acceptable for medical practitioners to send MCCDs to registration offices electronically and, in fact, this practice will form the foundations for the upcoming digitisation of the MCCD. The Cremation form 5 was not re-introduced after the Coronavirus Act expired and has been permanently removed.[10]

The temporary provision of allowing any medical practitioner to complete the MCCD, even if they did not attend the deceased during life, was discontinued and the process reverted to previous practice. Medical practitioners completing MCCDs must satisfy requirements set out in guidance around attendance and seeing the deceased.[11]

REFERENCES

1. NHS England. National Medical Examiner's Good Practice Guidelines, 2020. https://www.england.nhs.uk/wp-content/uploads/2020/08/National_Medical_Examiner_-_good_practice_guidelines.pdf (accessed 20 December 2021).
2. GOV.uk. Notification of Deaths Regulations, 2019. https://www.legislation.gov.uk/uksi/2019/1112/made (accessed 20 December 2021).
3. Ministry of Justice. Revised Guidance for Registered Medical Practitioners on the Notification of Deaths Regulations, 2020. https://assets.publishing.service.gov.uk/government/uploads/system/uploads/attachment_data/file/878083/revised-guidance-for-registered-medical-practitioners-on-the-notification-of-deaths-regulations.pdf (accessed 20 December 2021).
4. National Quality Board. Learning from Deaths, 2018. https://www.england.nhs.uk/wp-content/uploads/2018/08/learning-from-deaths-working-with-families-v2.pdf (accessed 20 December 2021)
5. Royal College of Pathologists. Cause of Death List, 2020. https://www.rcpath.org/uploads/assets/c16ae453-6c63-47ff-8c45fd2c56521ab9/G199-Cause-of-death-list.pdf (accessed 20 December 2021).
6. Office for National Statistics. Guidance for Doctors Completing Medical Certifications of Cause of Death in England and Wales, 2020. https://assets.publishing.service.gov.uk/government/uploads/system/uploads/attachment_data/file/877302/guidance-for-doctors-completing-medical-certificates-of-cause-of-death-covid-19.pdf (accessed 20 December 2021)
7. NHS England. National Exemplar – Administrative Information – Form ME-1 (Part A), 2018. https://www.england.nhs.uk/wp-content/uploads/2020/08/National_exemplar_-_administrative_information_ME1_A.pdf (accessed 20 December 2021).
8. NHS England. National Exemplar – Medical Examiner's Advice and Scrutiny – From ME-1 (Part B), 2018. https://www.england.nhs.uk/wp-content/uploads/2020/08/National_exemplar_-_advice_and_scrutiny_ME-1_Part_B.pdf (accessed 20 December 2021).
9. GOV.uk. Coronavirus Act, 2020. https://www.legislation.gov.uk/ukpga/2020/7/schedule/13/part/1/crossheading/medical-certificates-of-cause-of-death (accessed 20 December 2021).
10. England NHS UK. www.england.nhs.uk/coronavirus/publication/information-for-medical-practitioners-after-the-coronavirus-act-2020-expires/ (accessed 17 June 2022).
11. Gov.UK. www.gov.uk/government/publications/guidance-notes-for-completing-a-medical-certificate-of-cause-of-death (accessed 17 June 2022).

CHAPTER 5

The Role of the Medical Examiner Officer

Daisy Shale and Louise Parapanos

Medical Examiner Officers

Medical Examiner Officers (MEOs) are part of the Medical Examiner system (the term system is used in England, although in Wales, there is a single 'service'. (For the purposes of this chapter and elsewhere in this book, the acronym MES will be used interchangeably for both as the implications are similar). The MEO workforce supports and manages the MES and assists MEs with certain aspects of case scrutiny under delegated authority. The MEO's role is to support the ME with scrutiny and to ensure that a correct Medical Certificate of Cause of Death (MCCD) is issued to the bereaved, whilst identifying and passing on any areas of concerns with any aspects of an individual's care. Although MEOs are an integral part of the MES, they cannot work in isolation, or without suitable checks and review of their work. It is essential that there is no overlap or ambiguity between the roles of the ME and MEO. This also applies to those MEOs who undertake dual roles for a care provider such as an acute NHS trust, for example those who also work as a bereavement officer/advisor. The MEO cannot, and should not, replace the ME scrutiny (see Chapter 4) and cannot make the final decision on a case. It is also important to ensure that there is no unnecessary duplication of tasks, especially when it comes to the phone call to the bereaved. Roles and processes must be clearly understood within the individual MES team to ensure an efficient and effective service for the bereaved.

Under legislation originally proposed within the Coroners and Justice Act 2009, Part 1 Chapter 2 Section 19,[1] the ME must complete scrutiny of the clinical records and take an overview of all three components of scrutiny to determine the outcome of the case. This cannot be undertaken by the MEO, even in apparently straightforward cases. MEs can, however, delegate appropriate functions to the MEOs, allowing them to focus on the parts of the process that require ME input, facilitating the function of the ME office and minimising delays.

Workforce

The national model in the Implementing the National Medical Examiner's good practices guidelines[2] states that, for every 3000 deaths, there should be one whole time equivalent ME and three whole time equivalent MEOs. There are

Table 5.1   Examples of backgrounds from which the current England and Wales Medical Examiner Officers originate

• Anatomical pathology technologists	• Midwives
• Bereavement officers	• Mortality review
• Biomedical scientists	• Nurses
• Clinical audit and patient safety	• Operating department practitioners
• Coroner's officers	• Paramedics
• Counsellors	• Physician's associate
• Dieticians	• Police officers
• Lawyer/legal services	• Registrars
• Mental health services	• Teachers/education inspectors

approximately 540000 deaths per year in England and Wales, of which 490000 may be expected to be scrutinised by the MES. With the current workforce model and current death rates, the estimated MEO workforce in England and Wales will be around 450 whole time equivalent positions. Almost 400 individuals have completed MEO training.

It is important to remember that there is no set background for MEOs. On review of the current MEO workforce currently in England and Wales, not only have MEOs been recruited from the backgrounds usually associated with the bereaved, (e.g. bereavement officers or palliative care nurses), but also from a wide range of clinical, analytical, counselling, patient safety and other backgrounds. This diversity of skills, knowledge and experience has provided mutual support within the MEO workforce and networks established nationally, regionally and locally have driven the development of a close-knit and supportive new profession, in which every member can share their strengths and request support and guidance from their peers. Workshops, team meetings and professional groups have allowed MEOs to develop as a single workforce, to share good practice, and standardise systems and processes across the ME system.

Table 5.1 shows the range of experience of those in MEO posts in England and Wales.

The MEOs within a local MES may come from several of these backgrounds, dependent on the office set-up, number of deaths and any specialist areas associated with the ME Office. As for the ME, it is important that MEOs are individuals with empathy, a desire to learn, an enquiring mind, and excellent listening and communication skills.

The Team Approach

Healthcare as a whole has embraced the multi-disciplinary team (MDT) approach to medicine, recognising that every member of the team can add a different perspective to the group. MEOs are part of the MDT of death certification, and each may have a range of knowledge or skills that brings a different view to a case or may have ideas about a case that the ME or colleague MEO has not considered.

One of the key strengths of an MDT is that it avoids a single opinion or view and provides natural checks and balances within the team. If all aspects of case scrutiny are carried out by one single ME, mistakes or omissions are possible, and opportunities to discuss and learn from cases are missed. By delegating several of these tasks to the MEO team, the ME system creates its own internal safeguards and quality checks, whilst retaining its independence. The team or consensus approach ensures that the three components of scrutiny align to create an accurate reflection of the patient's last illness, including the reflections of those who delivered the care and the opinions of those who were present or knew the patient in life. It also facilitates learning and sharing of experience.

MEs can benefit from specialist knowledge and advice the MEO workforce can provide when considering complex or unfamiliar aspects of a case. MEs also come from a wide variety of clinical backgrounds and may have little (or no) experience in certain hospital specialties. Conversely, MEs from a hospital back-ground may have little community experience. MEOs can often give a different view on aspects of nursing care, intraoperative procedures, palliative medica-tions, feeding regimes or wound management, depending on their background. The broader and more diverse the background of MEOs and MEs in a team, the wider the knowledge base. This is of great advantage, taking a holistic view of care provided during the patient's last illness and allows a comprehensive review of all components of care received. In addition, MEOs from a non-clinical setting can also provide additional assistance in advising MEs and other stakeholders about roles such as death certification requirements, requirements for body dona-tion, consent to post-mortem examination and other processes relating to death certification as a whole.

This allows the local MES to provide information, guidance and assistance to all stakeholders of the service as required. It is vital to remember that the bereaved are at the heart of the service and that the process of death certification should be driven by the bereaved, and not be dependent on the ME's availability to under-take tasks which can otherwise be delegated.

Delegation of Work

The ME Services that have embraced the MEO role use a flexible approach to ensure that the bereaved and clinicians are provided with the most efficient deliv-ery of the service. This will take into account the different service models and staff groups within the teams and makes the best use of individual skill sets and knowledge for each individual case. In many ways, this is equivalent to a medical consultant responsible for patient care who has access to a support team of nurses, junior doctors, and other allied healthcare professionals to assist with the holistic management of their patients, or a Coroner responsible for investigating death who has access to a team of Coroner's officers, administrators, forensic pathologists and police officers to manage an investigation into death.

In more complex cases, the ME will speak to the clinical team and/or the bereaved to ask and answer questions about the patient's care, final illness and death. In more straightforward cases these tasks can be delegated to the MEO to undertake. As MEOs become more experienced, they are likely to take on a greater proportion of this work. An ME should always be available to speak to the doctor or family if they request it, or if the MEO feels it would be appropriate.

In other ME Services the MEO undertakes all delegatable tasks in every case and refers back to the ME if there are questions or concerns that require further clarity or consideration. ME teams must establish processes for cases in which the ME has not been able to complete scrutiny in the working day, and the MEO will complete any outstanding actions or discussions under delegated authority or arrange for another ME to complete the case.

For MEOs to be able to conduct these tasks they must have a clear understanding of the context of the case, they must be able to read and understand the medical records, and they must have an understanding of disease processes and medical and procedural terminology. It is essential that MEOs are able to understand and explain both the ME's and the clinical team's rationale and thoughts surrounding the cause of death accurately as well as explaining decisions made in relation to the patient's illnesses to both medical staff and the bereaved.

Documentation of any work undertaken by the MEO is vital – any conversations, decisions or outcomes must be recorded and should be identifiable to the individual MEO conducting the task, and by date and time. This information may be requested for legal proceedings, and so accuracy of recording is essential. The ME must satisfy themselves that tasks done under delegated authority have been satisfactorily completed by the MEO before confirming scrutiny has been completed. Any concerns raised by the bereaved or the attending team during conversations with the MEO must be discussed with the ME before agreeing on the next action.

These processes are broadly equivalent to those of the Coroner's officers, where the final decision regarding a case is made by the Coroner, but the gathering and collating of information, discussion with the clinical teams and the bereaved is done by the officers.

Benefits of the Medical Examiner Officer Workforce

Medical Examiner Officers are now established as part of the MES and are recognised as being integral to functioning of the service. As an emerging profession, there is a sense of pride in being responsible for continuity within the MES, by optimising ME time, assisting with preliminary case review or following up on missing information, performing actions under delegated authority and becoming the main point of contact for users of the service.

These benefits are perhaps most appreciated in cases in which there is a time-critical element such as a faith requirement for urgent release, or when other agencies are involved – such as organ donation or child deaths. The MEO can facilitate the scrutiny process to ensure all the components come together at the same time to enable a seamless process for the bereaved or the service users.

As MEOs are a constant presence in the office, they are ideally placed to carry out a range of functions including answering telephone enquiries, following up cases and referrals, collating information, accessing medical records, and tracking down missing information. They can also discuss cases with the qualified attending practitioner (QAP) and bereaved when they are ready to do so, without any time constraints or other pressures.

A well-trained and supported MEO workforce can manage multiple cases in various stages of completion, whilst handling several discussions, enquiries and new cases as they arrive. MEOs can also prioritise the service's workload, highlighting urgent cases to an ME. They can also ensure an ME's independence from the case, arrange a second ME review if required, and manage the office rota to ensure there is ME availability when and where needed.

Patterns and Trends

One of the benefits of the continuity provided by full-time MEOs is that they have an oversight of the service that enables them to identify trends within healthcare settings, whether related to communication issues, patterns in care, or concerns about medical or nursing care. With larger offices and multiple part-time MEs, patterns or trends may otherwise be missed. For example, an ME may pick up an issue with post-operative surgical infection on a certain ward, and so might several of the other MEs. Without the continuity provided by the MEO team, such trends may be missed. The MEO team can identify trends at local, regional and even cross-border level between England and Wales, as they can consider an overview of the cases reviewed by the MES as a whole, rather than just their individual case reviews. This real-time intelligence should be fed to the Lead ME to allow constructive feedback or act as the trigger to raise concerns with the care provider to drive change and improvement.

Training

With such a diverse range of individual skill sets, educating the MEO workforce and standardising processes and knowledge is paramount. For both MEs and

MEOs, the role is new and all will require training once in post (and where possible before). With the support of the Royal College of Pathologists, a complete programme of training has been developed, which consists of the same pathway as MEs through e-learning and face-to-face training. The face-to-face training day comprises of case discussion and information sessions with experienced MEOs, MEs, bereavement personnel, Coroner's officers and others, to facilitate the key aspects of the MEO role.

In addition to the e-learning and face-to-face training, a training portfolio for MEOs has been developed to provide guidance on required knowledge and skills, and to provide assurance to MEs and service users that the MEO team is appropriately trained to undertake delegated functions. Regionally and locally, there has been development of in-house training, information-sharing platforms and continuing professional development (CPD) programmes to ensure that those MEOs who require professional revalidation (for example, if they are from a nursing background), are able to do so. Learning is a continuous process for all those within an MES, and MEs and MEOs (both newly appointed and established) will need additional training, which may be via case discussions with MEs and other MEOs as well as more formal routes. In terms of MEO functions, the more training and education that is undertaken by MEOs, the more effective the MES as more tasks can be delegated with confidence.

For those MEOs who are from a clinical background, maintaining relevant registration is vital. The undertaking of CPD should be tailored to fit the role undertaken as MEO and to demonstrate ongoing competence of application of professional knowledge. It is also useful to look for additional training on topics such as end-of-life care, communication, disease process and treatment options.

Administration of Workload

Administration of the workload within the ME Office is crucial to ensuring effective and accurate documentation, independence, transparency and work flow. It is vital that all ME office functions are accurately documented in order to provide information to key stakeholders (Her Majesty's Coroner, registration services, bereavement offices, hospital trusts) and to allow for transparency and audit reporting.

There are several nationally approved documents created to help assist in the administration of workload. The first is the ME-1 (Part A) form (see Figure 2.2),[3] which was created to be used before any death documentation paperwork (MCCD, cremation papers) has been completed (see Figures 2.3 and 2.4). ME-1 (Part A) forms are also used to document the discussion between MEs/MEOs and the QAP. It is on this form that the QAP documents their proposed cause of death and indicates if they have any concerns regarding the patient's care or death. In practice, the ME-1 (Part A) form is not always utilised, but QAPs are encouraged to call or attend the ME office at a suitable time to discuss the circumstances of the case and talk through their proposed MCCD content. What is essential is that, prior to the ME/MEO discussion, the thoughts of the QAP are recorded to allow protection for the MES in such instances where, for example, it is alleged that the MEO has instructed the QAP as to what should be recorded as the cause of death.

This discussion is something that is often undertaken by the MEOs who, under delegated authority, discuss circumstances and causes of death with QAPs and, if necessary, can provide advice regarding the need for coronial notification. The member of the ME team who had the discussion with the QAP will then ensure this is documented using the ME-1 (Part B) form.[4] Many ME offices have adapted the exemplar ME-1B for local use and incorporated it into electronic mortality governance systems. This then allows the ME who is completing scrutiny of the case to be aware that a discussion has already taken place and whether any concerns were identified.

Some ME Offices have electronic systems that are part of NHS trusts' wider work on 'learning from deaths'.[5] At Norfolk and Norwich University Hospital for example, the Mortality Governance System houses completed structured judgement reviews (SJRs), minutes of morbidity and mortality meetings and local governance information, alongside the new and completed ME-1 (Part B)s. This system updates every 24 hours and shows a list of all deceased patients admitted to the mortuary overnight with all demographic information completed. This allows MEO review and ME scrutiny to be completed effectively and without delay. Although the MES ME-1Bs may be hosted on an in-house Mortality Governance System, access to and control of these data must be limited to the MES. However, it must also be noted that primary care and other community data must not be hosted on the system (see Chapter 12).

For other ME Offices covering cases from multiple trusts or care providers, a stand-alone system may be more practical than multiple systems linking into the multiple care providers' governance systems. Local discussion and agreement about access to MES data and information is crucial. For example, primary care data should not be recorded on hospital-based mortality governance systems.

At Norfolk and Norwich University Hospital, once the ME-1B has been completed on the system, and the whole case passed back through to the bereavement office, the case record is closed but can easily be searched for, should the information be required at a later date. Consideration of the ME-1 (Part B) being accessible to the care provider via the Mortality Governance System (MGS) to enable streamlined reporting is advised when setting up any local systems. The system allows the ME office to automatically escalate a case for an SJR or local governance, or raise a serious incident, and can also provide additional information that will help the reviewer, whilst restricting access to MES data to MES team members.

As part of the process by which the national ME service will become statutory, NHS Business Services Authority (NHSBSA) continues to make progress on the development of a digital solution for the MES. This is intended to provide a standardised system and will assist in the quarterly reporting currently done manually by all MESs. These data will be entered onto a web portal system, which collates the same set of data for every ME office, including total number of Coroner notifications and the outcomes, number of cremations/burials and the ethnicity of the deceased.

For the relevant information to be available for each office to submit the quarterly reporting, it is essential that the day-to-day workload of the MES is documented and easily accessible. The recording of this workload is undertaken primarily by MEOs, who are able to achieve this by virtue of being full-time in the office, and having complete oversight of the MES. As the national digital system is not yet available, every ME office makes its own decision on how best to collate and present these data. For example, at Norfolk and Norwich University Hospital these data are collated onto a Microsoft Excel spreadsheet, other offices use the RL Datix system (Wales), existing bereavement systems such as Ulysses (Sheffield) or bespoke data management systems. The data fields required in any system should align with the National data set included in the National Medical Examiner exemplar forms. As well as providing the figures required for the NHS England quarterly returns, this assists with internal office audit and feedback to the hospital Trust or Health Boards for research.

Thus, MEOs play a vital role in the administration of the overall MES. By ensuring accurate and accessible workload figures, the implementation and progression of this new service can be evaluated, and areas of learning identified.

Relationship between MEs and MEOs

The key to a successful and efficient ME office is to ensure that the working relationship between MEs and MEOs is open, honest and transparent. The differing roles between the two are clearly defined to ensure the smooth running of the service. It is at the discretion of the Lead or Senior ME to determine and satisfy themselves of the level of competency of the MEOs and to ensure that all parties are aware of their role within the MES. There may be some debate about the differences between an MEO with a clinical qualification and an MEO who has come from a non-clinical background. The NME National Good Practice Guidelines state that it is beneficial for MEOs to *'probably have experience in a patient or customer-facing role and of working in either current death certification systems, or a clinical or NHS setting . . . require an understanding of medical records and disease pathology . . . be able to provide advice on terminology and causes of death, and to explain these and the Medical Examiner's thoughts and rationale to Coroner's officers, doctors and those with no medical understanding . . . have strong interpersonal skills and be comfortable working with people following a bereavement'.*[2] This is important in order to be able to accurately advise and discuss causes of death and medical terminology, both with doctors completing paperwork and the bereaved.

The Lead or Senior ME has to be able to delegate several functions of the office to MEOs, which may include being the first point of call for all doctors within the care provider setting as well as other stakeholders, including registration and coronial services. Therefore having a clinical background equips the MEO with the ability to discuss potentially complicated medical terminology and situations with medical teams to ensure the MCCD is completed accurately and without delay. MEOs who have a clinical background may also be better placed to pick up different issues during the pre-review that may not be identified during the ME scrutiny. This ensures a well-rounded full scrutiny of the case to ensure all relevant information is captured, and if concerns are raised, is acted upon. MEOs from other backgrounds such as bereavement advisors and anatomical pathology technologists bring different but equally relevant perspectives and will be able to see the case from another perspective.

A professional and positive relationship between the ME and MEO is essential in order to ensure that open and respectful conversations are had in order to achieve the best outcome for the bereaved. Another benefit of having a good working relationship between all members of the MES is that, as the MEOs are the constant presence in the office, they can assist with new members of staff and visitors and help them familiarise themselves with the various processes and best ways of working. All members of the MES should feel comfortable asking questions to ensure a smooth process for the bereaved and to maintain a respectful working environment.

Challenges of the Role

The role of an MEO is extremely rewarding, although there are inevitably associated challenges. As the national Medical Examiner Office model is still not yet statutory, there can be challenges relating to establishing an MES. The main issue can relate to how best to embed the MES into already established mortality, bereavement and mortuary services. There have been some understandable concerns that the implementation of the MES would add another step to the process and cause associated delays for the bereaved and additional workload for clinical teams. The way these concerns can be overcome is to work closely with all relevant departments and teams, to ensure all are aware of the role of the MES, the safeguards it provides to both families and clinical teams and the importance of being an independent service. As the MES works alongside the hospital bereavement team and primary care administrative teams, this is a key area to focus on when developing a service. A strong joint working relationship needs to be established, placing the deceased patient and the bereaved at the centre of the service. All appropriate practices and policies should be discussed with relevant teams to ensure a smooth transition phase and an efficient working relationship. MEOs are vital in achieving and maintaining this relationship and, as the constant presence in the office, are ideally placed to ensure the smooth running of the whole MES.

Feedback from both bereaved families and clinical teams indicate that they find the opportunity to talk things through and discuss cases with an independent ME or MEO a positive experience. This helps to alleviate the initial concerns regarding the implementation of the new service.

Another area of initial difficulty is balancing the role of an independent service whilst working closely with mortality and quality and safety initiatives, to ensure all concerns captured are escalated appropriately. With a fully staffed and operational MES, and collaborative work with the Trust's or Health Board's medical and associate directors for quality and safety, and equivalent primary care colleagues, clear formal escalation plans can be created. A policy can then be created by the Lead MEO to ensure all members of the team are escalating concerns from the bereaved and staff in the correct and consistent way. This also ensures that the information gained from these concerns can be disseminated and any relevant learning shared.

This escalation process will be different for every acute trust and community setting in England, even when the MES becomes statutory. Wales has a single standardised approach to escalating concerns through the Once for Wales Mortality system. The independence of the MES must be maintained at all times; however, transparency must be achieved with the care provider in order to ensure that concerns and praise identified from scrutiny are handled appropriately. MEOs are best placed to advise other members of the MES on how best to escalate concerns or praise as, being the constant in the office, they are experienced with different scenarios.

The implementation and use of the Coronavirus Act (2020) regulations and legislation provided some challenges.[7] Before the Act came into force, there was more flexibility regarding meeting both families and medical teams face to face. Dependent on the state of the pandemic and on the local situation, death documentation may have been completed by the medical team on the wards and discussion with the bereaved took place on the telephone. Paradoxically perhaps, positive feedback has been common from bereaved families after a telephone call from the ME office, perhaps in part because it has simplified the process for them. The Coronavirus Act 2020 was time-limited legislation which expired in March 2022, but the Ministry of Justice and General Register Office (Home Office) have recently confirmed that the provision extending the requirement for having seen a deceased patient to 28 days, rather than 14 days prior to death, was made permanent through a change to regulations, and the government has indicated that Cremation Form 5 will not be re-introduced.[8] The provision for any medical practitioner to complete the MCCD, introduced as an emergency measure by the Coronavirus Act, was discontinued from 24 March 2022. It is yet to be seen, how the reversal of these easements affects the MES as a whole.

REFERENCES

1. GOV.uk. Coroners and Justice Act 2009. https://www.legislation.gov.uk/ukpga/2009/25/con tents (accessed 20 December 2021).
2. NHS England. Implementing the Medical Examiner System: National Medical Examiner's good practices guidelines, 2020. https://www.england.nhs.uk/wp-content/uploads/2020/08/ National_Medical_Examiner_-_good_practice_guidelines.pdf (accessed 20 December 2021).
3. NHS England. Administrative Information: Form ME-1 (Part A), 2018. https://www.england. nhs.uk/wp-content/uploads/2020/08/National_exemplar_-_administrative_information_ ME1_A.pdf (accessed 20 December 2021).
4. NHS England. Medical Examiner's Advice and Scrutiny Form ME-1 (Part B), 2018. https:// www.england.nhs.uk/wp-content/uploads/2020/08/National_exemplar_-_advice_and_scru tiny_ME-1_Part_B.pdf (accessed 20 December 2021).
5. National Quality Board. National Guidance on Learning from Deaths, 2017. https://www. england.nhs.uk/wp-content/uploads/2017/03/nqb-national-guidance-learning-from-deaths. pdf (accessed 20 December 2021).
6. NHS England. National Medical Examiner update, 2021. https://www.england.nhs.uk/ wp-content/uploads/2021/02/nme-bulletin-february-2021.pdf (accessed 20 December 2021).
7. Coronavirus Act 2020. https://www.legislation.gov.uk/ukpga/2020/7/contents/enacted? msclkid=47f37d4baf5e11eca52e2c6357ff2f0b
8. NHS England. National Medical Examiner update, 2022. https://www.england.nhs.uk/wp-content/uploads/2019/05/National-medical-examiner-bulletin-February-2022.pdf

CHAPTER 6

Completing a Medical Certificate of Cause of Death

Suzy Lishman and Jason Payne-James

Introduction

The Medical Certificate of Cause of Death (MCCD) is the certificate completed by a registered medical practitioner (doctor) who attended the deceased during their last illness and knows the cause of death. The MCCD is required for a death to be registered. Once registration has taken place, the registrar issues the death certificate, a certified copy of the entry in the register, which includes the cause of death provided by the certifying doctor. The registrar cannot amend the cause of death once the MCCD is written, including correcting spelling mistakes, so it is essential that the MCCD is completely fully and accurately.

Guidance about the completion of the MCCD is provided by the Office for National Statistics and HM Passport Office and is updated regularly. Since March 2020 until March 2022 guidance[1] took into account the easements of the Coronavirus Act 2020.[2] On 24 March 2022 the Act expired,[3] however some changes have been retained on a permanent basis, and other processes revert to previous practice. The following provisions continue:

- the period before death within which a doctor completing an MCCD (medical certificate of cause of death) should see a deceased patient will remain 28 days (prior to the pandemic, the limit was 14 days)
- it will still be acceptable for medical practitioners to send MCCDs to registrars electronically
- the Government's intention is that the form Cremation 5 (see Chapter 7) will not be re-introduced

The following emergency provisions changed with the expiry of the Act:

- the temporary provision allowing any medical practitioner to complete the MCCD will be discontinued
- informants will have to register deaths in person, not remotely.

The only requirement for the doctor completing the MCCD is that they attended the deceased during their last illness. There is no legal requirement to have seen

DOI: 10.1201/9781003188759-6

the patient in the 28 days before death or at any time after death. However, if a deceased patient has not been seen in the 28 days before or at any time after death, the registrar will automatically refer this to the Coroner if it has not already been referred by the attending doctor.

There is also general guidance at the front of each certificate book – the first four pages are notes for doctors and include instructions on how to complete the certificate. There are also short notes about when to refer to the Coroner and examples of industrial diseases on the back of each certificate.

Completing the MCCD is challenging but satisfying. A balance has to be struck between providing as much information as accurately and clearly as possible and in a sequence that explains what happened to the patient, while bearing in mind the sensibilities of the family and the rules by which registrars of births and deaths are governed.

Purpose of the MCCD

The MCCD has several purposes. It provides information to the family about the cause of death of their loved one, and allows them to register the death, proceed with funeral arrangements and settle the deceased's estate. The cause of death written on the MCCD provides a permanent record for generations to come – providing information about a family's health for immediate members and future genealogists. It also provides useful national statistics about causes of death, including informing future policy decisions about allocation of resources for healthcare.

Format of the MCCD

The MCCD is currently completed on paper by hand. Certificates are provided in a book by the registrar and must be kept securely at all times. A digital MCCD is being developed and is likely to replace the paper version in the next few years. The MCCD book includes a counterfoil, which remains in the book after the MCCD has been removed. A short version of the MCCD content is recorded on the counterfoil and retained by the general practice or hospital. Figure 6.1a and 6.1b show the front and reverse of a standard MCCD.

Before the implementation of the Coronavirus Act 2020, the completed MCCD was given to the informant in person, in a sealed envelope provided by the local registration service, and they would take it to the registrar. The Act provided for the completed MCCD to be scanned and sent electronically directly to the registrar. This easement has been retained since the expiry of the Act. The paper version is returned to the registrar in due course but is not required for registration of the death. This saves time and reduces the need for the informant to travel to collect the certificate. Following the expiry of the Coronavirus Act 2020, families must now register deaths in person, but do not need to provide the MCCD.

COUNTERFOIL

For use of Medical Practitioner, who should complete in all cases.

Name of deceased ....

Date of death ....

Age ....

Place of death ....

Last seen alive by me ....

Post-mortem/* Coroner 1 2 3 4

Whether seen after death* a b c

Cause of death:—

I (a) ....

(b) ....

(c) ....

II ....

Employment? ☐ *Please tick where applicable*

B. Further information offered?

....

Signature ....

Date ....

**Ring appropriate digit(s) and letter.*

BIRTHS AND DEATHS REGISTRATION ACT 1953

(Form prescribed by the Registration of Births and Deaths Regulations 1987)

MEDICAL CERTIFICATE OF CAUSE OF DEATH

For use only by a Registered Medical Practitioner WHO HAS BEEN IN ATTENDANCE during the deceased's last illness, and to be delivered by him forthwith to the Registrar of Births and Deaths.

Registrar to enter No. of Death Entry

Name of deceased ....

Date of death as stated to me .... day of .... Age as stated to me ....

Place of death ....

Last seen alive by me .... day of ....

1 The certified cause of death takes account of information obtained from post-mortem.
2 Information from post-mortem may be available later.
3 Post-mortem not being held.
4 I have reported this death to the Coroner for further action. *[See overleaf]*

Please ring appropriate digit(s) and letter

a Seen after death by me.
b Seen after death by another medical practitioner but not by me.
c Not seen after death by a medical practitioner.

CAUSE OF DEATH

The condition thought to be the 'Underlying Cause of Death' should appear in the lowest completed line of Part I.

	These particulars not to be entered in death register Approximate interval between onset and death
I (a) Disease or condition directly leading to death†	
(b) Other disease or condition, if any, leading to I(a)	
(c) Other disease or condition, if any, leading to I(b)	
II Other significant conditions CONTRIBUTING TO THE DEATH but not related to the disease or condition causing it.	

The death might have been due to or contributed to by the employment followed at some time by the deceased. ☐ Please tick where applicable

†This does not mean the mode of dying, such as heart failure, asphyxia, asthenia, etc: it means the disease, injury, or complication which caused death.

I hereby certify that I was in medical attendance during the above named deceased's last illness, and that the particulars and cause of death above written are true to the best of my knowledge and belief.

Signature .... Qualifications as registered by General Medical Council ....

Residence .... Date ....

For deaths in hospital: Please give the name of the consultant responsible for the above-named as a patient ....

(Form prescribed by the Registration of Births and Deaths Regulations 1987)

NOTICE TO INFORMANT

I hereby give notice that I have this day signed a medical certificate of cause of death of

....

Signature ....

Date ....

This notice is to be delivered by the informant to the registrar of births and deaths for the sub-district in which the death occurred.

The certifying medical practitioner must give this notice to the person who is qualified and liable to act as informant for the registration of death (see list overleaf). Where the informant intends giving information for the registration outside of the area where the death occurred, this notice may be handed to the informant's agent.

DUTIES OF INFORMANT

Failure to deliver this notice to the registrar renders the informant liable to prosecution. The death cannot be registered until the medical certificate has reached the registrar.

When the death is registered the informant must be prepared to give to the registrar the following particulars relating to the deceased:

1. The date and place of death.
2. The full name and surname (and the maiden surname if the deceased was a woman who had married).
3. The date and place of birth.
4. The occupation (and if applicable the name and occupation of the deceased's spouse or civil partner).
5. The usual address.
6. Whether the deceased was in receipt of a pension or allowance from public funds.
7. If the deceased was married or in a civil partnership, the date of birth of the surviving spouse or civil partner.

THE DECEASED'S MEDICAL CARD SHOULD BE DELIVERED TO THE REGISTRAR

Figure 6.1 (a) Front of Adult MCCD form.

PERSONS QUALIFIED AND LIABLE TO ACT AS INFORMANTS

The following persons are designated by the Births and Deaths Registration Act 1953 as qualified to give information concerning a death; in order of preference they are:

DEATHS IN HOUSES AND PUBLIC INSTITUTIONS

(1) A relative of the deceased, present at the death.

(2) A relative of the deceased, in attendance during the last illness.

(3) A relative of the deceased, residing or being in the sub-district where the death occurred.

(4) A person present at the death.

(5) The occupier* if he knew of the happening of the death.

(6) Any inmate if he knew of the happening of the death.

(7) The person causing the disposal of the body.

DEATHS NOT IN HOUSES OR DEAD BODIES FOUND

(1) Any relative of the deceased having knowledge of any of the particulars required to be registered.

(2) Any person present at the death.

(3) Any person who found the body.

(4) Any person in charge of the body.

(5) The person causing the disposal of the body.

*"Occupier" in relation to a public institution includes the governor, keeper, master, matron, superintendent, or other chief resident officer.

Complete where applicable

A

I have reported this death to the Coroner for further action.

Initials of certifying medical practitioner. ....

The death should be referred to the coroner if:

• the cause of death is unknown
• the deceased was not seen by the certifying doctor *either* after death *or* within the 14 days before death
• the death was violent or unnatural or was suspicious
• the death may be due to an accident (whenever it occurred)
• the death may be due to self-neglect or neglect by others

B

I may be in a position later to give, on application by the Registrar General, additional information as to the cause of death for the purpose of more precise statistical classification.

Initials of certifying medical practitioner. ....

• the death may be due to an industrial disease or related to the deceased's employment •
• the death may be due to an abortion
• the death occurred during an operation or before recovery from the effects of an anaesthetic
• the death may be a suicide
• the death occurred during or shortly after detention in police or prison custody

LIST OF SOME OF THE CATEGORIES OF DEATH WHICH MAY BE OF INDUSTRIAL ORIGIN

MALIGNANT DISEASES

	Causes include
(a) Skin	– radiation and sunlight
	– pitch or tar
	– mineral oils
(b) Nasal	– wood or leather work
	– nickel
(c) Lung	– asbestos
	– chromates
	– nickel
	– radiation
(d) Pleura and peritoneum	– asbestos
(e) Urinary tract	– benzidine
	– dyestuff manufacture
	– rubber manufacture
(f) Liver	– PVC manufacture
(g) Bone	– radiation
(h) Lymphatics and haematopoietic	– radiation
	– benzene

POISONING

(a) Metals	e.g. arsenic, cadmium, lead
(b) Chemicals	e.g. chlorine, benzene
(c) Solvents	e.g. trichloroethylene

INFECTIOUS DISEASES

(a) Anthrax

(b) Brucellosis

(c) Tuberculosis

(d) Leptospirosis

(e) Tetanus

(f) Rabies

(g) Viral hepatitis

	Causes include
	– imported bone, bonemeal, hide or fur
	– farming or veterinary
	– contact at work
	– farming, sewer or under-ground workers
	– farming or gardening
	– animal handling
	– contact at work

CHRONIC LUNG DISEASES

(a) Occupational asthma	– sensitising agent at work
	– farming
(b) Allergic alveolitis	
(c) Pneumoconiosis	– mining and quarrying
	– potteries
	– asbestos
(d) Chronic bronchitis and emphysema	– underground coal mining

NOTE:—The Practitioner, on signing the certificate, should complete, sign and date the Notice to the Informant, which should be detached and handed to the informant. Where the informant intends giving information for the registration outside of the area where the death occurred, the notice may be handed to the informant's agent. The Practitioner should then, without delay, deliver the certificate itself to the Registrar of Births and Deaths for the sub-district in which the death occurred. Envelopes for enclosing the certificates are supplied by the Registrar.

Figure 6.1 (b) Back of adult MCCD form.

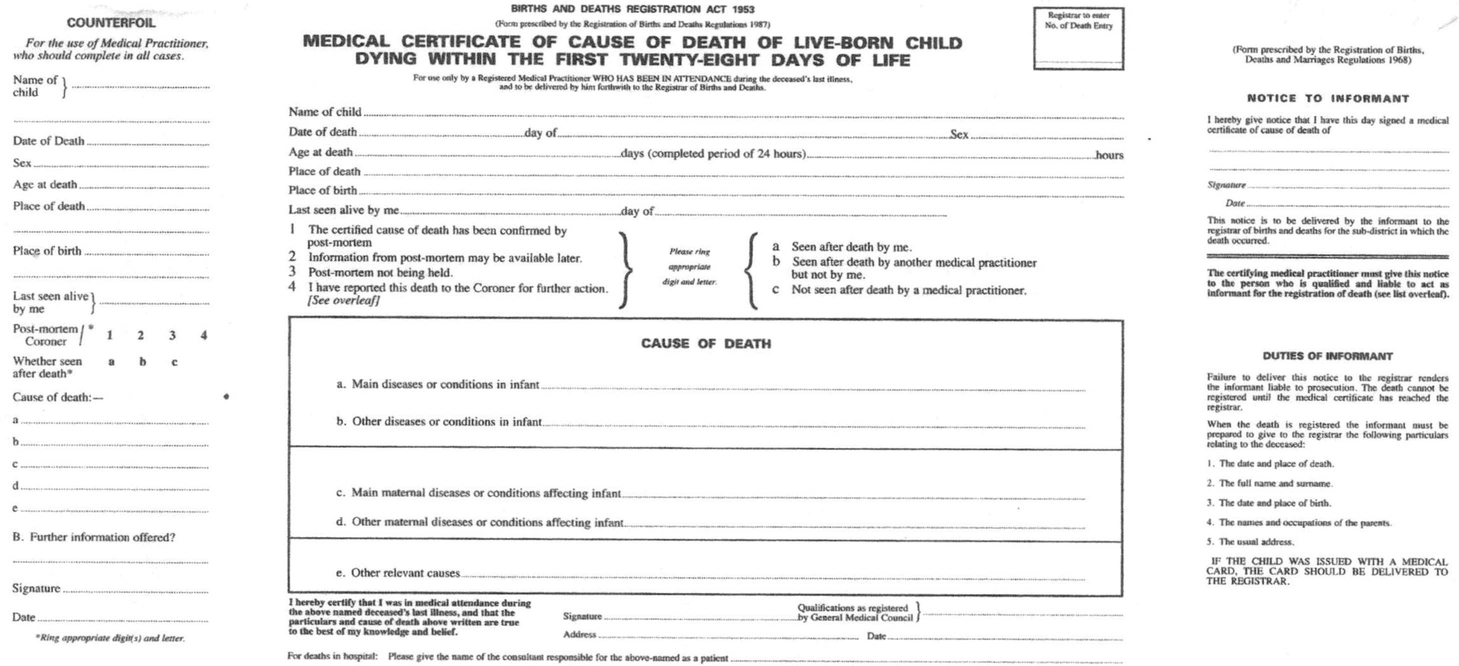
COUNTERFOIL

For the use of Medical Practitioner, who should complete in all cases.

Name of child } ....

Date of Death ....

Sex ....

Age at death ....

Place of death ....

Place of birth ....

Last seen alive by me } ....

Post-mortem / Coroner / * 1 2 3 4

Whether seen after death* a b c

Cause of death:—

a ....

b ....

c ....

d ....

e ....

B. Further information offered?

Signature ....

Date ....

**Ring appropriate digit(s) and letter.*

BIRTHS AND DEATHS REGISTRATION ACT 1953

(Form prescribed by the Registration of Births and Deaths Regulations 1987)

Registrar to enter No. of Death Entry

MEDICAL CERTIFICATE OF CAUSE OF DEATH OF LIVE-BORN CHILD DYING WITHIN THE FIRST TWENTY-EIGHT DAYS OF LIFE

For use only by a Registered Medical Practitioner WHO HAS BEEN IN ATTENDANCE during the deceased's last illness, and to be delivered by him forthwith to the Registrar of Births and Deaths.

Name of child ....

Date of death ....day of.................... Sex ....

Age at death ....days (completed period of 24 hours)....................hours

Place of death ....

Place of birth ....

Last seen alive by me....................day of....................

1 The certified cause of death has been confirmed by post-mortem
2 Information from post-mortem may be available later.
3 Post-mortem not being held.
4 I have reported this death to the Coroner for further action. *[See overleaf]*

Please ring appropriate digit and letter.

a Seen after death by me.
b Seen after death by another medical practitioner but not by me.
c Not seen after death by a medical practitioner.

CAUSE OF DEATH

a. Main diseases or conditions in infant ....

b. Other diseases or conditions in infant ....

c. Main maternal diseases or conditions affecting infant ....

d. Other maternal diseases or conditions affecting infant ....

e. Other relevant causes ....

I hereby certify that I was in medical attendance during the above named deceased's last illness, and that the particulars and cause of death above written are true to the best of my knowledge and belief.

Signature .... Qualifications as registered by General Medical Council } ....

Address .... Date ....

For deaths in hospital: Please give the name of the consultant responsible for the above-named as a patient ....

(Form prescribed by the Registration of Births, Deaths and Marriages Regulations 1968)

NOTICE TO INFORMANT

I hereby give notice that I have this day signed a medical certificate of cause of death of

....

Signature ....

Date ....

This notice is to be delivered by the informant to the registrar of births and deaths for the sub-district in which the death occurred.

The certifying medical practitioner must give this notice to the person who is qualified and liable to act as informant for the registration of death (see list overleaf).

DUTIES OF INFORMANT

Failure to deliver this notice to the registrar renders the informant liable to prosecution. The death cannot be registered until the medical certificate has reached the registrar.

When the death is registered the informant must be prepared to give to the registrar the following particulars relating to the deceased:

1. The date and place of death.
2. The full name and surname.
3. The date and place of birth.
4. The names and occupations of the parents.
5. The usual address.

IF THE CHILD WAS ISSUED WITH A MEDICAL CARD, THE CARD SHOULD BE DELIVERED TO THE REGISTRAR.

Figure 6.1 (c) Front of neonatal MCCD form.

Complete where applicable

A

I have reported this death to the Coroner for further action.

Initials of certifying medical practitioner. ....

B

I may be in a position later to give, on application by the Registrar General, additional information as to the cause of death for the purpose of more precise statistical classification.

Initials of certifying medical practitioner. ....

The Coroner needs to consider all cases where:

The death might have been due to or contributed to by a violent or unnatural cause (including an accident);

or   the cause of death cannot be identified;

or   the death might have been due to or contributed to by drugs, medicine, abortion or poison;

or   there is reason to believe that the death occurred during an operation or under or prior to complete recovery from an anaesthetic or arising subsequently out of an incident during an operation or an anaesthetic.

NOTE:—The Practitioner, on signing the certificate, should complete, sign and date the Notice to the Informant, which should be detached and handed to the Informant. The Practitioner should then, without delay, deliver the certificate itself to the Registrar of Births and Deaths for the sub-district in which the death occurred. Envelopes for enclosing the certificates are supplied by the Registrar.

Figure 6.1 (d)   Back of neonatal MCCD form.

Completion of the MCCD

Prior to the pandemic the MCCD had to be completed by a doctor who attended the deceased during their last illness and was able to provide the cause of death to the best of their knowledge and belief. Only a doctor can complete the MCCD; it cannot be delegated to a non-medical colleague, irrespective of their experience or status.

The emergency Act allowed any doctor who knew the cause of death to complete the MCCD in circumstances when the attending doctor is not available (for example because of illness, self-isolating or other clinical commitments). If the certifying doctor did not attend the deceased, they had to provide the name and General Medical Council (GMC) registration number of a doctor who did attend the deceased prior to death, or saw the body after death, on the MCCD. That easement ceased with the expiry of the Act and an MCCD can now only be completed by a doctor who attended the deceased during their last illness.

Attending during the last illness may be in person or by video consultation but not by audio only. An audio phone consultation is not an acceptable way of having 'attended' during the last illness. The certifying doctor, whether they attended the deceased or not, should have access to relevant medical records. Viewing a body after death, if it takes place, must be in person, not by video. There is no requirement for a body to be viewed after death if the person was seen alive by the certifying doctor (or another doctor) within the required time. The certifying doctor should usually have seen the deceased in the 28 days before their death.

The consultant who cared for a patient who dies in hospital is responsible for ensuring that the death is certified accurately and promptly, although they may delegate this to an appropriately trained and supervised member of their medical team. If a junior member of the team is tasked with completing the MCCD, they are encouraged to discuss the cause of death, and the wording used, with their consultant or another senior colleague before completing the certificate. Medical Examiners should discuss the wording of the MCCD with the certifying doctor (the qualified attending practitioner – QAP) after scrutinising the patient record, and they are ideally placed to advise on the most appropriate wording to be used.

Referring deaths to the Coroner

If no doctor saw the deceased in the 28 days before death or after death, the case must be notified to the Coroner.[4] Deaths must also be referred if the cause of death is not known, the death occurred in state detention, it was related to the deceased's occupation, or it may be due to unnatural causes. See Chapters 3 and 10 for further detail of coronial notification requirements.

Patient details

The MCCD includes a section for completion of the patient's details, including the full name, age, date and place of death. Care should be taken to ensure that all this information is correct, as it may cause difficulties for the family registering the death if any details are wrong. The registrar can correct any minor errors in this section of the certificate. The age should be given in years for anyone over the age of 1, and months if under one year. The name of the institution or private address where the patient died should be given. Deaths are usually registered in the district where they occurred, so it is important that the correct address is given.

Last seen alive

The MCCD asks when the deceased was last seen alive by the certifying doctor. The date should be given here, irrespective of whether another doctor has seen the deceased since. If the doctor completing the MCCD did not see the deceased alive, they should cross this out and write the name and GMC number of any doctor who did see the person alive. If the deceased was seen by video consultation this should be stated. A telephone consultation is not acceptable for this purpose.

Post-mortem examination

The certifying doctor must circle at least one of the four options given:

1. The certified cause of death takes account of information obtained from post-mortem
2. Information from post-mortem may be available later
3. Post-mortem not being held
4. I have reported this death to the Coroner for further action.

Option 1 is rarely circled as hospital (consented) post-mortem examinations are rarely performed in the UK nowadays, and if a coronial post-mortem has been performed the MCCD is not required.

Option 2 would usually only be circled if a hospital (consented) post-mortem is planned but has not yet taken place. If this is the case, the certifying doctor or the named consultant will receive a letter from the General Register Office (GRO) several weeks later asking if any further relevant information is available. An envelope is provided for the reply, which is sent directly to the GRO. If further information is likely to become available, the certifying doctor should initial section B on the back of the certificate to indicate that they may be able to provide additional information about the cause of death at a later date.

Option 3 is the option usually circled, as the majority of deaths where an MCCD is issued do not involve a post-mortem examination.

Option 4 is also commonly circled. If this option is selected, the certifying doctor must also initial section A on the reverse of the certificate to confirm that they have reported the death to the Coroner.

Seen after death

The certifying doctor must circle one of three options:

a) Seen after death by me
b) Seen after death by another medical practitioner but not by me
c) Not seen after death by a medical practitioner.

The above is self-explanatory. If the deceased was seen by another medical practitioner after death their name and General Medical Council (GMC) number should be recorded on the certificate. Medical practitioner here refers to a registered medical practitioner (doctor) and not any other healthcare professional. Death may be verified by an appropriately trained healthcare professional, such as a nurse or paramedic, but they cannot complete the MCCD.

Cause of death

The cause of death section is the most important section of the MCCD and the one that causes the most problems. There is a definite skill to formulating causes of death and not all doctors do it well. Medical Examiners (MEs) and some Medical Examiner Officers (MEOs) are trained in this area and play an important role in supporting certifying doctors in completing this section. It is important to understand that there may be a number of appropriate ways of expressing the same medical information. The ultimate responsibility for the cause of death given remains that of the certifying doctor (who records the cause of death to 'the best of their knowledge and belief'), so MEs and MEOs can guide but not insist on any particular wording. Registrars are not permitted to correct any spelling errors in this section so particular care should be taken to avoid mistakes. Words commonly misspelt include frailty (fraility is often written), and the 'a' is often missed out of the English spelling of words such as anaemia, ischaemia, septicaemia, and haemorrhage.

Format of cause of death

In the UK, the cause of death is written in the following form:

I(a) Disease or condition directly leading to death
I(b) Other disease or condition, if any, leading to I(a)
I(c) Other disease or condition, if any, leading to I(b)
II Other significant conditions contributing to the death but not related to the disease of condition causing it.

I(a) Disease or condition directly leading to death

The disease or condition directly leading to death is essentially the terminal event responsible for the death of the individual, such as gastrointestinal haemorrhage, acute myocardial infarction or pulmonary embolism. The mode of death should not be given here. Terms such as asphyxia, cardiac arrest, coma, exhaustion, organ failure, respiratory arrest, shock and syncope are not causes of death and are not required to be recorded. Occasionally recording a mode of death may be appropriate, but it must always be supported by an acceptable underlying cause of death in I(b). Adding terms such as 'chronic', 'terminal' or 'end-stage' does not make a mode of death acceptable.

The only organ failure that is now acceptable on its own is cardiac/heart failure. This should only be used in isolation if the underlying cause of the condition is not known. Ideally the cause should be given in I(b). Other organ failures (eg renal failure, liver failure, respiratory failure) are not acceptable as stand-alone causes of death.

It is entirely acceptable for a cause of death to consist of just I(a), with no further conditions on the MCCD. Examples include metastatic breast cancer, hypertensive heart disease or bronchopneumonia.

I(b) Other disease or condition, if any, leading to I(a)

However, many conditions that lead directly to death have an underlying cause. For example, upper gastrointestinal haemorrhage may be due to a gastric ulcer, an acute myocardial infarction may be secondary to long-standing ischaemic heart disease or coronary artery atherosclerosis, and pulmonary embolism may be due to clotting abnormalities brought about by an underlying lung cancer. The following would therefore be acceptable causes of death:

I(a) Upper gastrointestinal haemorrhage
 (b) Bleeding gastric ulcer

I(a) Acute myocardial infarction
 (b) Ischaemic heart disease

I(a) Pulmonary embolism
 (b) Squamous cell carcinoma of the left main bronchus.

I(c) other disease or condition, if any, leading to I(b)

Occasionally, a third step in the narrative of events leading to death is required. If an upper gastrointestinal bleed was due to bleeding oesophageal varices, for example, the underlying cause may be portal hypertension, cirrhosis or alcohol-related liver disease. In this case the cause of death could be given as:

I(a) Bleeding oesophageal varices
 (b) Portal hypertension
 (c) Cirrhosis.

What to do if there are more than three steps in the chain of events leading to death

It is often possible to omit the immediate cause of death without changing the accuracy of the MCCD, for example omitting respiratory failure, pulmonary oedema or haemorrhage, if the underlying cause is clear. It is also possible to include more than one condition on each line, for example:

I(a) Upper gastrointestinal haemorrhage from oesophageal varices (or just bleeding oesophageal varices)
 (b) Portal hypertension secondary to cirrhosis
 (c) Non-alcoholic fatty liver disease.

What if there is more than one cause of death?

If two conditions contributed directly to death, it is possible to include them both in one line on the MCCD and add (joint causes) after them. For example:

I(a) Congestive cardiac failure and chronic obstructive pulmonary disease (joint causes)
I(a) Cirrhosis
 (b) Chronic alcohol excess and hepatitis C infection (joint causes).

Part II

Part II of the cause of death is for conditions that have contributed to death but do not fit into the direct sequence described in part I. For example, diabetes mellitus may have contributed to deaths from ischaemic heart disease or stroke but is not a direct cause. Part II is not a dumping ground for every condition in the patient's past medical history. If a condition did not contribute to the death in any way, it should not be recorded on the MCCD.

Sense Check

When reviewing the cause of death, the condition in the lowest position in part I should be the underlying cause of death, i.e. the condition without which death would not have occurred. The sequence of events should read directly from lower to upper condition, i.e. I(c) caused I(b), which caused I(a). The conditions in I should not just be a random list of conditions, there should be a clear sequence. It can be considered as a reverse chronology, with I(a) being the most recent event.

Abbreviations

Abbreviations must be avoided on the MCCD. Some registrars will accept some abbreviations, but this varies and it is best practice to write everything in full, for example *Escherichia coli*, human immunodeficiency virus, chronic obstructive pulmonary disease rather than E.coli, HIV or COPD.

Possible/Probable

Possible and probable should not be used on the MCCD. The doctor completing the certificate provides the cause of death to the best of their knowledge and belief, so possible and probable should not be necessary and are likely to be rejected by the registrar. If a patient dies from disseminated malignancy, for example, and all the investigations so far have suggested a lung primary, but histological confirmation has not been obtained, it is perfectly acceptable to certify the death as being due to metastatic lung cancer. Writing 'metastatic cancer of probable/possible lung origin' is not necessary. If you really can't tell where the cancer has come from, 'disseminated malignancy of unknown origin' is an acceptable cause of death.

Accident/Injury

Terms such as cerebrovascular accident and acute kidney injury should ideally be avoided on the MCCD as they can cause confusion and distress for relatives, who may interpret them as suggesting that the deceased had an accident or was injured in some way. If they have been included, the ME or MEO can clarify this when contacting the bereaved family. However, alternative terms such as ischaemic stroke, right middle cerebral artery stroke or acute kidney disease avoid this problem.

Surgical and Medical Interventions

If any treatment has contributed to the patient's death, this should be included on the MCCD. However, this means that the registrar will reject the certificate unless the case has already been notified to the Coroner and a Form 100A issued. Interventions that have not contributed to death should not be recorded on the MCCD, as Coroner notification will still be required. If the terms 'operated', 'transplanted' or 'chemotherapy-related' are used, for example, Coroner referral will be required. Medical Examiners are particularly well placed to advise certifying doctors on this difficult area, and there may well be varying views from Coroners in different jurisdictions. Death due to neutropenic sepsis following chemotherapy for lymphoma, for example, may not usually need to be referred to the Coroner unless the treatment had been delayed or inappropriate, although some Coroners apply the guidelines more rigidly. Close communication with the local coronial team will ensure that appropriate notifications are made.

Going into Detail

You should provide as much detail as possible on the MCCD, including the cause of an infection, if known, and the type and site of origin of any malignancy. For example:

I(a) *Proteus mirabilis* urinary tract infection
I(a) *Streptococcus pneumoniae* pneumonia
I(a) Squamous cell carcinoma of the left main bronchus
I(a) Metastatic goblet cell adenocarcinoma of the appendix.

Deaths from SARS-CoV-2 Infection

Deaths from COVID-19 are often a direct result of pneumonia, in which case 'COVID-19 pneumonia' is an entirely acceptable stand-alone cause of death. However, many patients with COVID-19 infection have involvement of several organ systems. In such cases, 'COVID-19 infection' would be more appropriate. It is also known that many underlying conditions increase the likelihood of an individual dying from COVID-19 infection. As these conditions didn't lead directly to death, but predisposed to the poor outcome, they should be listed in part II of the cause of death. Examples include hypertension, type 2 diabetes mellitus, immunodeficiency (state the cause if known), underlying malignancy (include the type), chronic lung conditions such as chronic obstructive pulmonary disease, cystic fibrosis or asthma, sickle cell disease or stage 5 kidney disease.

Just because someone dies following a positive SARS-CoV-2 PCR test, it obviously doesn't mean that it was necessarily cause of death. Careful consideration should be given to the contribution of COVID-19 infection to the patient's death, including it in part I only if it was directly responsible for the death, part II if it was a contributory factor, and not at all if infection did not contribute to death.

Cause of Death List

An acceptable cause of death is one that the registrar can register without referring to the Coroner. There is no definitive list of every acceptable cause of death; however, the Royal College of Pathologists published the Cause of Death List[5] in 2020 to clarify some of the questions most often raised by certifying doctors and registrars. The list is extremely useful, but some gaps and anomalies remain, and it is currently being updated. A revised version is expected in 2023. Registrars of births and deaths are not medically qualified and cannot use their discretion to decide whether a cause of death is acceptable or not. Some proposed causes of death are obviously not acceptable – those that only give a mode rather than a cause of death and deaths that are clearly unnatural, such as those following an accident, assault or poisoning.

There are also conditions that may be related to the individual's occupation, such as mesothelioma or pneumoconiosis. If such a death is definitely not related to the deceased's occupation, 'non-occupational' should be added to the cause of death to ensure that the registrar does not reject it.

There are conditions that could be traumatic, so it should be made clear if they are not, such as including 'spontaneous' before intracranial haemorrhage.

Table 6.1 gives some examples of the guidance provided in the Cause of Death List.

Old age/frailty/senility

Old age, frailty and senility (and variants) should only be used when no more specific cause can be given, and the deceased was over 80 years old. Death from old age is usually preceded by gradual deterioration over weeks, months or years. If a death is sudden, 'old age' is rarely appropriate, irrespective of the age of the deceased.

Interval between onset and death

To the right of the cause of death is a box asking how long each condition was present. The immediate cause may be precisely dated, such as following a stroke or

Table 6.1   Examples of the guidance provided in the Cause of Death List[4]

Instruction	Example
Acceptable	Chest infection, congestive cardiac failure, coronavirus infection, dementia, dissection of thoracic aorta, ischaemic heart disease
Refer to Coroner	Anaphylaxis, cryptogenic fibrosing alveolitis, dehydration, haemothorax, hypothermia, iatrogenic, injury, malnutrition
Refer to Coroner unless supported by another acceptable condition	Cardiac arrhythmia, aspiration pneumonia, cardiac tamponade, general debility, haematemesis, hypoxic brain injury, jaundice
Refer to Coroner unless doctor states non-industrial	Angiosarcoma of liver, anthracosis, brucellosis, mesothelioma, pneumoconiosis, silicosis
Refer to Coroner if may be linked to the deceased's occupation	Bladder cancer, lung cancer, emphysema, hepatitis, pulmonary tuberculosis
Acceptable if deceased over 80	Old age, debility of old age, frailty of old age
Acceptable if qualified as spontaneous or with an acceptable underlying cause	Bowel obstruction, gastrointestinal bleed, intracerebral haemorrhage
Not acceptable as a standalone cause of death	Depression, hypertension, learning disability, gastric ulcer
Refer to Coroner unless doctors states it was caused by an underlying disease	Fracture

acute myocardial infarction. It is acceptable to indicate that underlying conditions have been present for 'months' or 'years'. This section is not recorded on the death certificate and is often not completed by the certifying doctor.

Death related to employment

Under the cause of death box the certifying doctor is asked to tick a box (sometimes referred to as the 'Spearing box', after Nigel Spearing MP, who introduced the Industrial Diseases (Notification) Bill in 1981) if *'the death might have been due to or contributed to by the employment followed at some time by the deceased.'* This should be considered in all cases and the deceased's previous occupations should be sought if a cause of death may be employment-related. If this box is ticked the case must be referred to the Coroner as the registrar will be unable to register it.

Certifying doctor

The final section of the certificate is the signature and qualification of the certifying doctor. The doctor's name should be printed in block capitals in addition to the signature and the registered qualifications and GMC number given. The residence is usually given as the hospital or GP practice where the doctor is based. For hospital deaths the name of the consultant responsible for care of the patient must also be provided.

Table 6.2 provides a checklist to identify whether the MCCD has been properly completed.

Table 6.2a   Completing the MCCD – a checklist

- Has every section been completed?
- If 2 or 4 have been circled, has the back of the certificate been initialled?
- Has the name and GMC number of a doctor who saw the deceased during the last 28 days, or after death, been included?
- Does the sequence of cause of death make sense?
- Does part II only contain conditions that contributed to death?
- Are all of the conditions listed acceptable (see Cause of Death List)?
- Has the possibility of an occupationally acquired condition been considered?
- Is the form signed and dated, and the GMC number of the doctor provided?
- Has the stub been completed?

Table 6.2b   Key points to avoid registration delays

DO NOT USE:	DO PROVIDE:
• Abbreviations	• Cause and site of infection
• Modes of death	• Type and primary site of cancer
• Possible/probable	• 'Non-industrial' where appropriate
• Natural causes	• 'Spontaneous' where appropriate

Stillbirths and Deaths of Live-born Children Dying within the First 28 Days of Life

The standard MCCD should not be used for recording the deaths of stillborn children or deaths within the first 28 days of life. There is a separate Certificate of Still-birth and Neonatal Death Certificate for these deaths (see Figure 6.1c and d). Stillbirths are infants born after 24 weeks gestation that did not show any sign of life after being born. Any child that has breathed after birth is regarded as a live birth, irrespective of the gestation.

The Future of the MCCD

Plans are underway to replace the current paper MCCD with a digitised version. This will make completion and transmission easier. It also provides an opportunity to add new fields to the certificate, such as the ethnicity of the deceased.[5] Once the ME system is statutory, the ME will review and approve all digital MCCDs, essentially adding their 'stamp' to indicate that they have scrutinised the case, just as some MEs currently stamp the paper certificate.

REFERENCES

1. Office for National Statistics. Guidance for doctors completing Medical Certificates of Cause of Death in England and Wales, 2020. https://assets.publishing.service.gov.uk/government/uploads/system/uploads/attachment_data/file/877302/guidance-for-doctors-completing-medical-certificates-of-cause-of-death-covid-19.pdf (accessed 31 March 2022).
2. GOV.uk. Coronavirus Act, 2020. https://www.legislation.gov.uk/ukpga/2020/7/contents/enacted (accessed 31 March 2022).
3. NHS England. Coronavirus Act expiry. Death certification and registration; easements from 25 March 2022. March 2022
4. GOV.uk. The Notification of Death Regulations, 2019. https://www.legislation.gov.uk/uksi/2019/1112/made (accessed 20 December 2021).
5. The Royal College of Pathologists. Cause of Death List, 2020. https://www.rcpath.org/uploads/assets/c16ae453-6c63-47ff-8c45fd2c56521ab9/G199-Cause-of-death-list.pdf (accessed 20 December 2021).
6. House of Commons. Women and Equalities Committee. Unequal impact? Coronavirus and BAME people, 2020. https://committees.parliament.uk/publications/3965/documents/39887/default/ (accessed 20 December 2021).

CHAPTER 7

Basics of Law for Medical Examiners and Medical Examiner Officers

Nigel Callaghan and Gabriel Callaghan

A Very Brief Introduction to the Law

This section of the chapter provides a general background of how the legal system in England and Wales works. Scotland and Northern Ireland have their own legal systems.

How is law made?

England is a common law jurisdiction, meaning that judges can make law by precedent in a judgement that binds other decisions by judges. Common law is essentially 'judge-made' law. Judges in the lower courts must follow the precedent of another court when deciding cases. These laws are not 'codified', i.e they are not written down in an Act. Murder is a common law offence.

Other laws are created by Acts of Parliament, such as the Coronavirus Act 2020. This Act gave the power to ministers to create statutory instruments, such as activating a lockdown. Acts of Parliament are voted on by MPs in the House of Commons, and in the House of Lords.

The courts

Courts are divided into criminal and civil jurisdictions.

Criminal courts hear matters that negatively affect society as a whole. Criminal prosecutions are brought by the Crown Prosecution Service (CPS) on behalf of the Crown when there is a public interest to prosecute, and there is a reasonable prospect of a conviction. Rarely, a private prosecution is brought that does not involve the CPS. Criminal offences can be summary (those that a magistrates' court can deal with) or indictable (those that can only be dealt with in a Crown court). Manslaughter by gross negligence and fraud are examples of criminal offences that may be committed in a medical setting.

DOI: 10.1201/9781003188759-7

Civil courts handle legal disputes that are not necessarily crimes, for example personal injury, clinical negligence litigation and other claims for compensation. In civil cases there is no 'prosecution' by the 'Crown'. Rather, the claimant, who can be a person, group, business, institution or government body, brings a claim of harm against the respondent.

The High Court of Justice typically hears actions in complex cases and claims for high financial sums, such as those involving clinical negligence. County courts hear claims for lower financial amounts. These courts typically do not sit with a jury.

The high court has jurisdiction to hear judicial reviews, for example challenges to the procedures that a public body (e.g. the General Medical Council – GMC) has used to make a decision. The three grounds for judicial review are: illegality, which is defined as a body not having a legal power to make a decision; procedural unfairness if there is evidence of bias; and irrationality, which is a decision that no reasonable person should have made. An added ground is if the procedure breaches the Human Rights Act. If the judicial review is successful, the decision is quashed. Examples of judicial reviews are decisions where an NHS trust has issued a 'do not resuscitate' order without appropriate consultation with a family, or treatment is refused by a trust.

Coronial courts involve a Coroner sitting to determine the cause of death. The coronial system is discussed in Chapter 10.

The burden of proof

There are two standards of proof in English law, depending on whether it is a civil or criminal matter. In the criminal courts, the standard of proof is 'beyond reasonable doubt', sometimes expressed as 'satisfied so that you are sure', which means being sure of guilt. An example of when this test would not be satisfied is when there is a convincing alibi. In the civil courts, the test is 'on the balance of probabilities' (i.e. whether it is more likely than not to have occurred).

Hearsay evidence in English law

A Medical Examiner (ME) may be privy to 'hearsay evidence', for example 'Doctor X said that he heard Doctor Y comment about Patient Z'. There are rules regarding the admissibility and weighting of hearsay evidence.

Hearsay evidence is admissible in the Coroner's court, but the Coroner must consider what weight to attach to the evidence; or, if it's a jury inquest, the Coroner must direct the jury to consider what weight to attach to it.[1] The Civil Evidence

Act 1995 states that hearsay evidence is admissible in the civil courts, but the lawyers are required to serve the evidence on the other party, and they can apply to prevent this. The rules in the criminal courts are stricter under the Criminal Procedure Rules 2020; a notice of hearsay evidence is required to be served on the court officer by the party wishing to rely on it, and each of the other parties is served a copy. The judge determines admissibility when it is in the interests of justice to allow a particular piece of hearsay evidence.

Human Rights and Equality Law

Religious and cultural requirements surrounding the ME system are explored in Chapter 15. In this section, the law relating to equality and human rights is discussed.

The Equality Act 2010 states that no person must be discriminated against (either directly or indirectly) based on the following protected characteristics: age, gender reassignment, being married or in a civil partnership, being pregnant or on maternity leave, disability, race including colour, nationality, ethnic or national origin, religion or belief, sex and sexual orientation. UK human rights law is covered by the Human Rights Act 1998, although considerable political discourse surrounds this. The most relevant sections in terms of the role of the ME are Article 2, which requires an independent investigation when a person dies in circumstances that involve the state, and Article 9, which details freedom of thought and religion.

The ME system is new, and at the time of writing, there have been no court cases testing the implications of the system on the Human Rights Act. However, a source of authority can be found from cases involving the Coroner's office. One case tested the right enshrined in Article 9. This case concerned delays in a Coroner ordering a non-invasive CT scan for a member of the Jewish faith, to determine whether a conventional post-mortem examination was required.[2] In the Jewish faith, there is a requirement for burial to occur within 24 hours of death as a sign of respect to the deceased; however, in this case this did not happen due to delays. The Coroner in this case implemented a 'cab rank' rule, which did not account for religious needs. It was ruled that the rule was unlawful since it did not adequately account for faith requirements, and it was not compatible with human rights law.

A guidance note produced by the Chief Coroner stated that there is no obligation to give automatic priority, but *'Coroners should pay appropriate respect to the faith of the deceased'.*[3] A Medical Examiner Service (MES) may encounter the issue as described in this case and it is therefore suggested that there will be a legal obligation to consider the faith requirements of any deceased person, and the implications of any actions or inactions by the MES.

A second case involved an Orthodox Jew who died in the Royal Free Hospital after a brief illness.[4] Jewish law forbids the desecration of a corpse via post-mortem examination if at all possible, so the family offered to pay privately for a CT scan.

The Coroner refused this request, instead requiring a conventional post-mortem examination. The family were dissatisfied, so they obtained a high court injunction preventing the post-mortem until the matter could be resolved. It was ruled by the court that the CT scan could have allowed the Coroner to establish the cause of death, and that the Coroner was wrong and had not adequately considered the human rights implications.

Confidentiality and Data Protection

Confidentiality is a fundamental tenet of professional ethics. Breaching confidentiality can damage trust in the medical profession. Indeed, a data protection breach, such as death records being left visible to the public on a desk or people discussing a death in a public area, could cause substantial harm if a vulnerable relative finds out about a death from the 'grapevine'.

There are obligations described in the General Medical Council's 'Good Medical Practice'[5] relating to the confidentiality of the medical records of deceased persons, which are stricter than the Data Protection Act. A doctor still owes a duty of confidentiality to patients after their death, although the doctor must also promote and protect the health of patients. To facilitate this requirement, there are a limited number of circumstances in which a doctor can disclose identifiable information. These are shown in Table 7.1.

When disclosing data to an external person or organisation, a doctor should only disclose the information required to achieve the purpose; for example, it may not be necessary to disclose all of the medical records of a patient. Under the Access to Health Records Act 1990, anyone who may have a claim resulting from the person's death can apply to have access to the medical records of a deceased person. Disclosing all of the medical records may cause distress to the family; for example, a patient may have had a sexually transmitted infection they don't want their family to know about. All doctors should be mindful of this.

Table 7.1 Examples of circumstances in which a doctor can disclose identifiable patient information

- The disclosure is required by law, e.g. a court order, or by the Coroner
- The patient gave informed consent before death
- The disclosure is required to prevent harm to others, e.g. a safeguarding issue arises
- A body has a statutory power to request the data, e.g. the Care Quality Commission or the NHS Business Fraud unit
- The disclosure is in the public interest, e.g. for public health reasons

Table 7.2 Examples of scenarios that qualify for protected disclosures

- A criminal offence has been committed, is being committed or is likely to be committed
- A person has failed, is failing or is likely to fail to comply with any legal obligation to which they are subject
- The health and safety of any individual has been, is being or is likely to be endangered
- Information tending to show that one of the above matters is being, has been or is likely to be concealed

If an ME is unsure about anything related to data protection, they should consult the Caldicott Guardian in their organisation. Generally, if disclosing patient information, an ME should be prepared to explain and justify the decision.

Public interest disclosures – Whistleblowing

An ME may have a 'reasonable belief' that serious failings have occurred and that patients were put at risk, or someone may disclose this to the ME. MEs are ideally placed to receive such disclosures because of the independence of the role. In this instance a 'public interest disclosure' is made, as defined in the Public Interest Disclosure Act 1998, allowing the matter to be drawn to the attention of someone other than the ME's employer if necessary. Table 7.2 shows examples of scenarios that qualify for protected disclosures.

A 'protected disclosure' can be made to an ME's employer, a legal adviser or a 'prescribed person', which includes regulatory bodies such as the General Medical Council and the Care Quality Commission. To qualify for protection, the disclosure must be made in good faith and not for personal gain. Legally, any confidentiality clause that prevents a practitioner from making these disclosures is void.

There is a legal and professional duty of candour for health care professionals to notify when an incident occurs that causes harm or distress, or the incident has the potential to do so.

Professional Negligence

Professional negligence is a notoriously complex subject. Negligence is a civil matter covered under the 'law of torts'. Professional negligence occurs when a medical practitioner has breached the legal duty of care attributed to a skilled and competent practitioner, harm has been caused by the breach, and the damage was not remote from the negligent act (i.e the damage must be foreseeable by a competent doctor). In this section, this definition is explored further.

An ME may not be involved with bringing or defending legal actions for negligence, but it is useful to have an idea of the legal tests when reviewing deaths in the ME role, to determine whether the death was attributable to staff failings.

Duty of care

Legally, a breach of a duty of care and therefore negligence (obligation to not act or fail to act in any way that results in harm) is defined in case law,[6] with the tripartite test being:

1. The harm must be reasonably foreseeable.
2. There must be a reasonable degree of proximity between the claimant and defendant (e.g., a doctor treating a patient).
3. It must be fair and just to impose a duty of care.

The standard of care is that of a reasonable and competent medical practitioner, following generally accepted professional practice, such as recommended by the National Institute for Health and Care Excellence (NICE). A junior doctor is required to perform to the standard of a competent and skilled doctor working in the same post, *impurities culpae ad numerator* ('Ignorance, or want of skill, is considered a negligence, for which one who professes skill is responsible'). For example, you would expect any doctor to be competent in cardiopulmonary resuscitation (CPR) and taking blood, regardless of seniority. However, if the doctor is a consultant or has specialist skills, then they are held to the standard of a person holding those skills above a less qualified doctor.

It is not only clinical staff who owe a duty of care. A 2018 Supreme Court case concerned a man who had sustained a head injury after an assault and went to the emergency department.[7] The receptionist told him there would be a five-hour wait to see a doctor, which was inaccurate. As a result, the man went home, and developed traumatic brain injury. The court ruled that the traumatic brain injury probably would not have occurred if the man had stayed in the emergency department, and he would have stayed if he had been told an accurate waiting time.

Proximity and causation

For a legal action related to negligence to be successful, there needs to be sufficient closeness to the events of the action, and its consequences. The test is, 'but for the negligent action, would the consequence have been avoided?' An example would be a doctor not recognising obvious warning signs of sepsis, after which the patient died but would not have died if the obvious signs had been recognised.

However, 'causation' in the legal sense can be complex. Case law surrounds the 'remoteness of damage'. One judgement considers the hypothetical case of a doctor who examines a mountaineer's knee, and negligently pronounces the knee fit.[8] The mountaineer goes climbing, which they wouldn't have done if the knee had been pronounced unfit, and suffers an injury from an avalanche unrelated to the knee. The House of Lords ruled that it would be unreasonable to assume that 'proximity' occurs in this situation as the causation was too remote, and the 'avalanche' could not be reasonably foreseeable.

Generally, the test is based on the balance of probabilities (a likelihood of 51% or more); is it more likely than not that the negligence caused the death, or made it occur sooner than anticipated? One case involved a general practitioner (GP) failing to diagnose a malignant melanoma in the claimant's groin after an examination.[9] The court found that the lack of diagnosis would have reduced the claimant's life expectancy by three years, so the court found the GP liable.

Another case surrounded a patient who was examined by a doctor for Driving and Vehicle Licencing Agency (DVLA) purposes due to high blood pressure.[10] The patient died nine years later from a stroke, and the doctor was charged with failing to send a letter to the patient's GP. The court ruled that negligence could not be proved as there was no basis for finding that it was probable that the stroke was caused by the failure to treat hypertension, so causation was not established.

Examples of negligence judgements

One case involved doctors being held negligent for diagnosing a child with tonsillitis, when the child actually had meningitis.[11] The patient was on intramuscular antibiotics, which had the effect of masking the symptoms of meningitis as tonsillitis. Later, the patient acquired cerebral palsy due to the misdiagnosis. The court ruled that the doctor was negligent since a reasonable and competent doctor would have noticed that the patient was on intramuscular antibiotics and would have considered a meningitis diagnosis.

Conversely, another case ruled that a GP was not negligent in not referring a baby to hospital for meningitis, although the baby was later admitted to hospital and diagnosed with meningitis.[12] The GP was not held liable because the evidence disclosed at the time would not have led a reasonable and competent GP to make a diagnosis of meningitis.

Unusual circumstances have to be accounted for in determining negligence. One set of proceedings involved a patient who had surgery to reverse an ileostomy, but later suffered complications and had to have their colon removed.[13] The patient had a unusual anatomy. Negligence was not proven in this case since the claimant's anatomy would make it particularly easy for damage to be done, so it could not be said that the standard of the surgeon fell below the standard of a reasonable and competent surgeon.

Criminal Law

The purpose of this section is not to criminalise doctors for making an honest mistake. The purpose is to identify conduct of a criminal nature that could put patients at risk and instances where further action must be taken to prevent a recurrence of harm.

Dishonesty

The legal test surrounding dishonesty before 2017 was defined by the Ghosh Test, which was a subjective test in which the defendant themselves must have appreciated that their conduct was dishonest, such as submitting a false timesheet.[14] However, the Ghosh Test was updated with the objective Ivey Test in 2017 by the Supreme Court, which stated that the Ghosh Test did not correctly represent the law.[15] The Ghosh Test could yield some absurd results, in the sense that it stated that the defendant themselves had to appreciate that what they were doing was dishonest by the ordinary standards of reasonable people. Under that test, the defendant would need to be acquitted if they did not think what they were doing was dishonest. The Ivey Test for dishonesty is:

1. What was the defendant's actual state of knowledge or belief about the facts?
2. Was the defendant's conduct dishonest by the standards of ordinary decent people?

Thus, someone is dishonest if the decent 'man on the street' would view their conduct as dishonest.

Fraud

At a high level, fraud is defined as knowingly misrepresenting or concealing the truth with an intent to cause a gain for someone, or to cause another person loss. Fraud can be committed by making a false representation, abuse of position or failure to disclose information, i.e. in an insurance contract. For fraud to occur via false representation, a defendant must dishonestly make a false representation with an intent to make a gain for themselves or another. Examples of fraud in the medical setting would be a doctor being dishonest about their qualifications or experience to obtain employment or submitting invoices for consultations that never occurred.

Conspiracy to pervert the course of justice

Conspiracy to pervert the course of justice is a common law offence that potentially carries a sentence of imprisonment for up to life. The offence occurs when a person does a series of acts (inaction is not enough for the offence) that have a tendency to obstruct justice (i.e. cover something up). The 'course of justice' starts after an investigable event occurs, for example after a death for which a doctor is responsible. Examples of obstructions include falsifying medical records to cover up manslaughter by gross negligence, persuading a witness to alter the evidence they give and concealing or destroying evidence (e.g. knowingly destroying a blood sample or medical records). Withholding evidence that would prove the innocence of a doctor would be covered by this offence.

Offences against the person

Battery is a common law offence under English law. Battery is a form of assault that requires the unlawful and non-consensual application of force.[16] There are various forms of assault covered by the Offences against the Person Act 1861, such as actual bodily harm and grievous bodily harm (defined as very serious bodily harm such as broken limbs). Wounding can occur when the skin is broken. There have been examples of medical staff who have assaulted patients, such as at Winterbourne View Hospital, where patients were slapped and assaulted by the staff.

Ill-treatment or wilful neglect

Ill-treatment and wilful neglect are criminal offences of the Criminal Justice and Courts Act 2015. The Act was born out of the events occurring at the Mid Staffordshire NHS Trust. Before these offences were introduced, it was already an offence under the Mental Capacity Act 2005 to ill-treat or neglect patients who lacked capacity; however, the new Act makes it an offence to ill-treat or neglect a patient who has capacity.

In this Act, 'wilful' means that an action was deliberate or reckless as opposed to a genuine accident. Being reckless can include an attitude of not caring. Examples of 'wilful neglect' include withholding medication. Ill-treatment actions have the potential effect of degrading the dignity of a patient.

Murder, manslaughter and corporate manslaughter

Murder can occur in the medical setting and is the offence for which Harold Shipman, whose actions have been so significant in the creation of the ME system, was convicted. For a murder to be proven, there needs to be an intention to kill or to cause grievous bodily harm. The defendant must have foresight that a consequence of their actions is the potential to cause death. Causation is discussed in the section on 'professional negligence'. An example of murder in a hospital setting would be administering a noxious substance or a fatal dose of a drug to a patient, with the intent to kill them. Murder does not necessarily require a person to make a fatal blow, such as stabbing a victim to death. Under the law of 'joint enterprise', anyone assisting in a murder, knowing the likely consequence of their act, for example supplying the chemicals for murder, could also be found guilty of murder.

Manslaughter occurs where a death was unintentional, but the defendant intentionally carried out an unlawful and dangerous act from which death inadvertently resulted. A dangerous act occurs when a 'sober and reasonable' bystander would deem it as such. Manslaughter by gross negligence is a challenging offence to prove, but it occurs where a healthcare professional breached a duty of care causing death, and the breach has to be so grossly bad that it deserves to be treated as a crime.[17] This is a higher standard than negligence. *R v Khan* involved a surgeon who was convicted for a 'catastrophic mistake' in administering a toxic dose of anaesthetics.[18]

Corporate manslaughter can be committed by an NHS trust or care provider, where the company does something grossly negligent that occasions a death. In one collapsed case against an NHS trust, Mr Justice Coulson stated that corporate manslaughter requires negligence to be so truly bad that it warrants criminal liability.[19] A theoretical example of circumstances occasioning a charge would be management recklessly short-staffing an intensive care unit to such a level that it was dangerous.

Currently, both assisted suicide and euthanasia are criminal offences in England and Wales, with euthanasia being prosecuted as either murder or manslaughter, although there is political and ethical debate around this at the time of writing. Assisted suicide is helping someone to commit suicide either by providing drugs knowing what they are going to be used for or procuring travel to another jurisdiction for euthanasia. A murder prosecution could occur when someone administers a fatal dose of a drug with the intent of ending a life, despite having the intent of killing the person to end their suffering. It is important to note that withdrawing life support when there is no reasonable prospect of recovery is typically not a criminal offence.

REFERENCES

1. Thornton QC. Law Sheet No. 4. Hearsay Evidence, 2014. https://www.judiciary.uk/wp-content/uploads/2020/08/law-sheets-no-4-hearsay-evidence.pdf (accessed 20 December 2021).
2. Royal Courts of Justice. Adath Yisroel Burial Society & Anor, R (On the Application Of) v HM Senior Coroner for Inner North London, 2018. https://www.judiciary.uk/wp-content/uploads/2018/04/aybs-v-hmcoroner-judgment.pdf (accessed 20 December 2021).
3. Lucraft QC. Guidance Note 28 – Report of Death to the Coroner: Decision Making and Expedited Decisions, 2018. https://www.judiciary.uk/wp-content/uploads/2020/08/guidance-no-28-report-of-death-to-the-coroner-2010517.pdf (accessed 20 December 2021).
4. Royal Courts of Justice. R (on the application of Rotsztein) v HM Senior Coroner for Inner North London, 2015. https://www.judiciary.uk/wp-content/uploads/2015/12/r-rotsztein-v-hm-senior-coroner-for-inner-london-2015-ewhc-2764-admin.pdf (accessed 20 December 2021).
5. General Medical Council. Good Medical Practice, 2019. https://www.gmc-uk.org/ethical-guidance/ethical-guidance-for-doctors/good-medical-practice?msclkid=19c7bee0af6711ecac3d3a1bc4ca8cdf
6. Caparo Industries plc v Dickman. UKLH 2, 1990.

7. Darnley v Croydon Health Services NHS Trust. UKSC 50, 2018.
8. South Australia Asset Management Corp v York Montague Ltd. UKHL 10, 1996.
9. JD v Mather. EWHC 3063 (QB), 2012.
10. Sims v MacLennan. EWHC 2739 (QB), 2015.
11. SC v University Hospital Southampton NHS Foundation Trust. EWHC 1610 (QB), 2020.
12. Doy v Dr Gunn. EWHC 3344 (QB) 2011.
13. Saunders v Central Manchester University Hospitals NHS Foundation Trust. EWHC 343 (QB), 2018.
14. R v Ghosh. EWCA Crim 2, 1982.
15. Ivey v Genting Casinos (UK) (trading as Cockfords Club). UKSC 67, 2017.
16. R v Afolabi. EWHC 2960, 2017.
17. R v Rudling. EWCA Crim 741, 2016.
18. *Manchester Evening News*. Hospital doctor killed dad-of-four after giving him lethal anaesthetic overdose before 'routine' procedure, 2020. https://www.manchestereveningnews.co.uk/news/greater-manchester-news/hospital-doctor-killed-dad-four-19257819 (accessed 20 December 2021).
19. R v Cornish and another. EWHC 2967 (QB), 2015.

CHAPTER 8

Role of the Bereavement Service

Meryl Hepple

Introduction

There is an overlap between the function of a bereavement service and a Medical Examiner Service (MES). The role of the bereavement team (BT) varies from hospital to hospital, but the fundamental aims remain the same. From the perspective of the BT, the introduction of the Medical Examiner (ME) has added a welcome additional layer of scrutiny to the service. Initial concerns about encroachment on jobs have been allayed and clarification about the roles of the two services has enabled great collaboration and mutual support. The introduction of the new MES in 2019, followed the next year by the COVID-19 pandemic, placed substantial pressures on individuals and teams. The pandemic has brought about the greatest change to the practical aspects of the work of the BT. Some of these changes have persisted following expiry of the Coronavirus Act 2020 and others remain and some will hopefully revert back in due course. Face-to-face registration has returned but the completed Medical Certificate of Cause of Death (MCCD) is scanned to the registration office, Cremation Form 5 no longer being required, and any belongings being handed over to the funeral director (FD) when they collect the patient.

Role and Activities of a Bereavement Team

The role of the bereavement team (BT) is to support the next of kin with the practical and emotional aspects of registering the death, making funeral arrangements and retrieving personal effects. The BT coordinates the everyday, administrative and legal processes and bereavement advisors (BAs), also known as bereavement services officers (BSOs), are the key contact point between doctors, Medical Examiners (MEs) and Medical Examiner Officers (MEOs), mortuary, ward staff, Coroner's office, funeral directors and next of kin. BAs gather appropriate information from the family/informant and make sure they understand what to expect and the time frame involved. As soon as a doctor has completed the death documentation and the MES has undertaken the scrutiny, the family can proceed with registering the death and the patient can be released to the funeral director.

The first contact with family is the most important because the BT are gathering crucial information such as the occupation of the deceased, the name of the funeral director and whether the deceased is to be buried or cremated. A BA builds trust with the next of kin and helps them to understand what is expected from them in terms of contacting the funeral director, when and how they are going to register the death as well as receiving and paying for certificates, and the expected time frame within which their loved one can be released from the mortuary and into the care of the funeral directors. This conversation takes place in a way that allows them to share their experience or emotions and was particularly important during lockdown when families were not able to be at the bedside when their loved one was at the end of life. There may be other events going on in their lives such as family disputes or complex situations at home, or another relative in hospital, or that they are feeling lonely and lost without their significant other. The BAs consider it a privilege to be able to listen, empathise and be the main point of contact, and these first conversations usually take around 10 to 15 minutes depending on the circumstances of each individual. BTs believe that the time spent with the next of kin will free up valuable time for the MES, doctors or Coroners so that they can concentrate on the medical and medicolegal aspects of the case.

Specific Case Types

Many deaths are not straightforward so BAs are trained in matters such as organ or body donation, repatriation, specific religious or other funeral arrangements (some of these may need to be referred to the Coroner's office and not all cases have a satisfactory outcome). Equally, the family unit is often complex and determining who will take responsibility for the funeral is often far from clear.

Perhaps the patient died in the emergency department and the general practitioner (GP) hadn't seen them recently, or they died at home within days of a hospital discharge. Perhaps the responsibility for death documentation falls to a doctor who looked after the patient out of hours and is not available due to shift patterns, moving jobs or illness. These are examples of situations that occur often and the BT identifies and contacts the appropriate doctor to remind them to speak to the MES before writing the MCCD. For out-of-hospital deaths that occurred following a recent discharge, liaison may be made with the Coroner's office, unless the patient was discharged for palliative care and the hospital team is able to complete the paperwork.

The workflow may be most efficiently managed by holding a team brief each morning to bring the BAs up to speed with relevant events, discuss an action plan for outstanding cases, determine priorities and assign new deaths among the team. Any deceased patients who wished for their body to be donated or had other specific wishes such as repatriation or urgent funerals on religious grounds are taken into consideration when prioritising the workload. The death of a baby is assigned to an advisor or bereavement manager with additional specialist training.

The Approach of the Bereavement Team

The BT does everything it can to take the pressure off clinical and ward staff, and provide practical and emotional support to doctors, families, mortuary, ward staff, Coroners and legal services.

Any relevant information received regarding the care of the patient in hospital, as well as comments made about the care leading up to the admission, should be documented. At the Norfolk and Norwich Hospital this is done on our software system and can be accessed by the MES. Bereavement advisors do not specifically ask about concerns, but if the family volunteers positive or negative comments about treatment, this is documented. The BAs explain to all bereaved families that the hospital has a Medical Examiner Service and any concerns can be raised with them when they receive the routine MES call. Advising the family to expect the call from the MES is important, giving them the opportunity to think about any questions they might have, and ensuring that they are not alarmed when they receive the phone call. If any urgent concerns are raised, these are brought to the attention of the MEO team, who will discuss them with the ME.

Often the family divide responsibilities during and after the patient's life, and the ME may speak to a different person from the BA. For example, one relative may have been the main carer (and have knowledge of the medical history) and another sibling could be arranging the funeral and registering the death, either as executor or by mutual agreement within the family. When the bereavement team is made aware of these complexities, clear instructions from the family are documented and the MES informed. Close collaboration between the services and a constant two-way flow of information allows both MES and BT to optimise the efficiency of their work, avoid duplication and enhance the effectiveness of the service given by the two teams.

Release of Patients

When the MES has completed the appropriate paperwork, the BT calls the relatives to explain they can register the death and confirm funeral arrangements. In Norwich the funeral directors are emailed with a clearance reference number so that they can collect the deceased without waiting for the death to be registered. The cremation papers are sent to the mortuary for the funeral director to collect along with the patient and any belongings they have with them. Each hospital will have different processes for the release of bodies and sharing of cremation forms.

Contract Funerals

For situations where there is no money, no provision made for a funeral or a reluctance of family to pay, the team makes extensive searches to establish the financial viability for a funeral. Additional searches are carried out if the deceased has no family.

If nobody comes forward the hospital has a contract price with a local funeral director and the hospital is obliged to arrange and pay for the funeral. This involves the death being registered by the manager or deputy bereavement manager, in their role as applicant for the funeral arrangements, cremation, and the ashes being scattered at the local crematorium. The funeral is paid for by the trust, but in the event that there is no known family, or funds being tied up in the deceased's estate, work continues with financial and legal institutions, including Treasury Solicitors and the local council, in an effort to recoup the funeral costs. The Human Tissue Act 2004 only allows the mortuary to hold the deceased for a maximum of 30 days, after which it is necessary to freeze the body. With many mortuaries having limited capacity, BTs should be mindful of the 30-day rule and endeavour to ensure the funeral has taken place by then.

Administration, Communication and IT Systems

In addition to day-to-day contact with mortuary, Coroner's office, doctors and MES, enquiries are processed from a huge variety of individuals and bodies including social services, council offices, solicitors, GPs, department of anatomy, registration service, crematoriums, medical secretaries, ward clerks, PALS and complaints. Additionally, if a hospital colleague suffers a personal bereavement, either at the hospital or in the community, there is always a BA ready to listen and provide practical and empathetic support.

Communication is the most important part of the bereavement services role and this may be done via a combination of telephone calls, emails and electronic means. Most hospitals will have an in-house mortuary database that is used as the main communication board for deceased patients, with authorised staff being able to read and add key information. There may be a separate mortality governance system and the MES will, of course, collect its own information.

During the pandemic, although face-to-face meetings with families ceased, if relatives arrived at the hospital reception desk and asked to speak to a BA, the BA would arrange to see them in a quiet space, while observing COVID-19 protocols.

Babies

The death of babies requires different processes. The hospital chaplains (or other faith representatives) may go through funeral options with the family. The parents are asked to sign a funeral preference form and they receive a copy of this, together with appropriate advice and contact details. Many parents ask for a post-mortem examination or may have been advised to have genetic testing when their baby dies, and in these cases a specialist bereavement midwife is able to provide the appropriate clinical and practical support to the doctors, midwives and parents regarding any consents required. This approach is effective; it ensures informed consent regarding the funeral wishes of the parents and chaplains are able to spend time with grieving parents as well as providing pastoral care.

The processing of guiding bereaved parents through the completion of the paperwork required following the death of a baby requires specialist training and this is a key element of the role for senior BAs. Such BAs need to be trained to recognise the forms needed at each trimester and to check that the correct papers are completed in accordance with the gestation, circumstances and funeral wishes. Mistakes or omissions (sometimes by clinicians) are corrected before sending to the mortuary. The MES will scrutinise all neonatal deaths, based on a collaborative approach with the neonatologists and paediatricians. The BT liaises with the MES to have sight of the papers for scrutiny before sending the neonatal MCCD to the registration service. For stillbirths and non-viable foetuses the advisor makes sure that the correct death documents have been completed and any stillbirth certificates are sent to the registration service as quickly as possible to prevent further distress to the parents. Stillbirths do not currently fall under the remit of the MES, although there is a campaign by bereaved families and stillbirth charities for this to happen.

Some FDs have particular skills with younger deaths, but those FDs who don't usually deal with baby deaths often benefit from the guidance and reassurance of the BT.

Doctors, Coroner Notifications and Outcomes

Whilst doctors should complete MCCDs or notifications by the end of their shift, two working days are allowed locally before there is an escalation process, which is followed to avoid unnecessary delays. The BT works closely with ward staff to achieve this.

Once the doctor who is going to complete the paperwork has been identified, they are contacted and the urgency of the task is explained. The BT reinforces the MES message that they should speak to their consultant to agree a proposed cause of death before discussing it with the MES.

Doctors are expected to call the next of kin if they are making a Coroner referral and explain the reason for the referral, and this must be done in good time. BAs can provide non-clinical support and advice about what else they might need to do. Many doctors have only completed a few coronial notifications and some none at all. This is another area where the BT and MES roles overlaps and both can support the clinical teams and the bereaved families by expediting and explaining the process.

Families often find this process daunting; the bereavement advisors offer reassurance and answer any general non-clinical questions that the family have (e.g. 'I was told that the Coroner is involved. What happens next?' 'Will this delay the funeral?' 'Should I tell the funeral directors?' 'When can I register the death?' 'What happens to my uncle's belongings?).

If the doctor is able to write or amend MCCD and cremation paperwork with a Coroner's reference, the BT will update the MES and contact the certifying doctor to finish the papers as a priority. The family are updated on the timescale for registering the death and when their loved one can be taken into the care of the FD.

If there is to be a post-mortem examination, the medical records are sent to the mortuary for the pathologist and, if there is an inquest, the Coroner's team takes over arrangements with the family, the bereavement office updates their records and the medical records are tracked out to clinical coding.

Interim Measures during COVID-19

The COVID-19 pandemic impacted on BT workload by increasing the number of deaths, resulting in delays to the completion of paperwork in many cases. In Norwich, the MES felt it appropriate that attending doctors should continue to complete death documentation. This was done on the wards to avoid any cross-contamination in the bereavement office. Discussion about causes of death was done remotely. The doctor would complete the appropriate paperwork and contact the bereavement office for support regarding non-clinical questions for the completion of relevant forms. In other MESs, the ME took over completion of the MCCD following discussion with the attending doctor and agreement about the cause of death. This arrangement meant that doctors did not need to attend the bereavement office and the BT did not need to enter wards, thus minimising the risk of infection. It also freed up busy frontline doctors to care for patients.

The BT has seen an improvement in attitude toward the completion of death documentation, which may be down to the joint BT/MES induction training and awareness programme, which should be mandatory in any hospital.

Easements during the pandemic

The practice of scanning MCCDs to the registration service which commenced in the pandemic and has been retained since the expiry of the Coronavirus

Act 2020 in March 2022 works well. Initially, some families were upset that they were not able to meet with a BA and register the death in person. However, many families, particularly those who live some distance away, appreciated being able to complete registration of the death without having to travel to the hospital to collect the MCCD.

Conclusions

BAs put the family first and everything is centred on making this a smooth process, which is delivered as quickly as possible so that the death can be registered within five days and the patient can be taken into the care of the funeral directors.

Some junior doctors find the cremation forms time-consuming and intimidating. Doctors used to spend around 15 minutes to complete death documentation (which included a telephone referral to the Coroner that was supported by a reference and subsequent paperwork, or a decision to refer to Coroner). They now spend about 30 minutes completing the MCCD, cremation documentation and the death notification and/or a Coroner referral on the ICE computer system. This doesn't include a discussion with the consultant for an agreed cause of death (assuming that they are on duty at the same time and that the consultant has seen the patient) then a further discussion with the MES prior to completing the appropriate paperwork.

Cremation fees do not provide sufficient incentive for many doctors to complete cremation papers.

As the population has increased and the hospital is constantly under severe pressure, it adds to the challenge of locating an appropriate doctor with sufficient knowledge of the patient to agree a proposed cause of death with the consultant and the ME, then complete the appropriate death documentation.

When the MES was first introduced we found that this extra layer of scrutiny was a seamless service and it was clear from the outset that it would add value. Although the scrutiny of community deaths will not directly affect our team, we appreciate the significant impact on their workload.

The Future

With the introduction of the Medical Examiner Service, it may be time to review the Births and Deaths Registration Act of 1953 in England and Wales, which states that deaths should be registered within five (calendar) days (including weekends and bank holidays). This is particularly challenging if the patient dies on a Friday evening because the following Monday is classed as day four in registration terms, but only day one in the hospital setting. Perhaps this could be amended to fall in line with Scotland's law of registering a death within five working days.

Whatever the changes, they should be directed towards improving support of the bereaved whilst enhancing patient safety and identifying vulnerabilities and risks.

CHAPTER 9

The Role of the Registration Officer (Registrar)

Deborah Smith

Introduction

Delivery of civil registration services in England and Wales is the joint responsibility of the General Register Office (GRO) and local authorities (LAs). GRO is part of Her Majesty's Passport Office (HMPO), a directorate of the Home Office (HO).

GRO was founded with the passing of the Births and Deaths Registration Act of 1836.[1] This legislation required that a registrar should formally record details of births and deaths in England and Wales; in Scotland and Northern Ireland it is slightly different. Prior to that, Church of England parish records were the only source of registration, but this meant that the increasingly non-conformist population was not being correctly recorded. Additionally, as the post-industrial revolution workers migrated to cramped city conditions, a clearer means of obtaining causes-of-death statistics and mortality rates generally was needed.

The legislation has been refined and reformed over the succeeding years to meet the changing needs of the population. Current legislation is provided by the Births and Registration Death Act 1953.[2] It is a statutory duty to register births and deaths.

Today, registrars are the employees of their local authority but they work under the ruling and guidance of GRO.

What Is a Registrar?

A registrar's duty is to record legally the details of births and deaths that have taken place in their sub-district in a register held for this purpose. The registrar can also issue and certify copies of these register entries when purchased by the appropriate parties. It is the registrar's duty to ensure that these certificates are only issued to those who are entitled to possess this information, in accordance with the legislation.

DOI: 10.1201/9781003188759-9

The registrar is responsible for the safety and security of the register and for all documentation relating to it. They collect, record, reconcile and bank all relevant fees.

Registrars also conduct and record civil partnerships and civil (and some non-conformist) marriages and maintain the corresponding records. They ensure that due legal process is followed in the taking of notices of intention to marry or form a civil partnership; particularly in checking documentation and interviewing the parties concerned; occasionally referring notices to GRO or the Home Office. The paperwork for marriages taking place in Church of England churches is usually dealt with by the clerical incumbent.

A registrar also has to perform numerous administrative tasks relating to registrations such as facilitating the re-registrations of births after marriages or civil partnerships have been formed, carrying out corrections to registers, ensuring that birth and death appointments are booked in good time and generally helping the public with their enquiries.

To become a registrar, you need to have an understanding of, and respect for, the laws that govern registration. You need to be able to combine task efficiency with compassion for the people with whom you are dealing. Registrars engage with the public at the most crucial and emotionally turbulent moments of their lives: when they marry or form a civil partnership, when their children are born, when their family members die. There is no higher praise for a registrar than to hear the words (particularly after a death registration): 'Thank you – you have made that so much easier for me.'

As the law changes all the time, so does civil registration, so registrars need to be able to keep up with these developments and undertake further training as appropriate. For instance, the information in this chapter is correct at the time of publication but it is subject to change.

For example, some registrars worked from home during the COVID-19 pandemic but the nature of most types of registration and the security surrounding the documentation of them, meant that many needed to work in offices. These offices have been adapted for further personal protection of both the public and the staff. Amongst other additional tasks, this has meant that registrars have to clean desks, chairs and equipment between public-facing appointments.

Registration of Death

A death that has taken place in England and Wales must be registered within five calendar days of its occurrence and in the district in which it happened. In Scotland, registration must take place within five working days, which reduces some of the time pressures that are present in England and Wales. The five-day

Table 9.1 Individuals qualified to be an informant (17(2) of the Births and Deaths Registration Act 1953)

(2) The following persons shall be qualified to give information concerning the death, that is to say—
(a) any relative of the deceased who has knowledge of any of the particulars required to be registered concerning the death;
(b) any person present at the death;
(c) the occupier of the property where the person died
(d) any person causing the disposal of the body.

requirement is one that may cause much concern to next of kin, who often require reassurance that they will not be penalised if for reasons out of their control the 'rule' is breached. Although individuals are highly unlikely to be penalised, the five-day requirement is one of the parameters by which registration office performance may be measured.

To register the death, the registrar must be in possession of a correctly completed Medical Certificate of Cause of Death (MCCD). It is the registrar's duty to ensure this certificate is in order before registration begins and also that the person who wishes to register the death qualifies as an informant. This would normally mean that they would be a relative but there are other criteria that would enable someone to be a qualified informant, such as arranging the funeral. Table 9.1 (taken from the s17(2) of the Births and Deaths Registration Act 1953) provides details of who an informant for death registration might be.

Checking an MCCD

There are many checks a registrar must do on an MCCD. If a doctor has not completed it correctly, it wastes the registrar's time while they contact the surgery or hospital to check and could also result in an appointment being wasted and further distress being caused to relatives. Chapter 6 provides information on how best to complete an MCCD.

Registration Challenges Arising from Anomalies and Omissions on MCCDs

Date of death not corresponding with information given by informant

The deceased's name and the place and date of their death is legally provided to the registrar by the informant, rather than the doctor. However, if a doctor has confirmed a date for a person's death on an MCCD that differs from when the informant said they died, this can cause problems with arranging the funeral, particularly in relation to cremation paperwork. For example, sometimes confusion may arise if a death occurred shortly before midnight, but was not verified until after midnight (i.e. on the following day).

'Last seen alive by me' date too long ago or omitted

The doctor *must* provide a 'last seen alive by me' date and circle (1), (2), (3) or (4) (usually '(3) Post-mortem not being held') and must also circle 'a) Seen after death by me', 'b) Seen after death by another medical practitioner but not by me' or 'c) Not seen after death by a medical practitioner'.

If b) or c) have been circled, the certifying doctor must have seen the patient within 28 days of death.

Causes of death reportable or abbreviated

The registrar must check that the causes of death are permissible according to the Cause of Death List published by the Royal College of Pathologists and the local Coroner's Cause of Death list.[3]

If any causes of death are unacceptable or the registrar is in any doubt about how one might lead to another, then the registrar must contact a Coroner's officer to verify them. Ultimately, it is the responsibility of the registrar to ensure that the causes of death they are registering are acceptable. The Coroner's officer might give the registrar the go-ahead or they might ask them to refer the death to the Coroner's office, which can be done on an electronic form, on paper or via a portal. The registrar would then have to take some details from the informant for the referral, explain that the registration could not go ahead and submit the information for the Coroner's consideration.

A referral to the Coroner can also be triggered by the informant giving the registrar information that may not have been available to the doctor, such as suspicions that the death was industrial-related or that the deceased suffered mistreatment or neglect either by themselves or others. This should happen less as Medical Examiners scrutinise more deaths and families have the opportunity to discuss any concerns prior to registration.

Additionally, most abbreviations are not permitted in the causes of death recorded on MCCDs. Registrars are not medically-trained and therefore must record exactly what the doctor has written on the MCCD including abbreviations and spelling mistakes, even if the doctor has explained them. This can result in the MCCD being amended or a new certificate having to be issued for clarity which, in turn, results in more delay.

Any occasion when a registrar has to contact a doctor's surgery or hospital constitutes a delay to the appointment and a waste of time and resources. This can be further exacerbated if the certifying doctor is not at work for any length of time.

Signature, qualifications, GMC number, residence and date of completion omitted or unclear

The MCCD must be signed (with the doctor's name printed next to it) and dated by the doctor and their qualifications and the General Medical Council (GMC) number must be written on it, together with the name of the surgery or hospital to which they are attached.

This is so the registrar can access the GMC website in order to check that the doctor is licensed to practise and record this fact, together with the doctor's name and primary qualification in pencil on the MCCD. The death cannot be registered without the doctor providing this information for the registrar to check.

Carrying out the Registration

Once all the checks have been satisfactorily carried out, the registrar then combines the personal information about the deceased (such as date and place of birth) provided by the informant, with the medical information provided by the doctor. This information is entered into an online registration system, which generates the register page for signing by the informant and the registrar.

Paperwork Issued after Registration

The registrar takes payment for any certified copies of the register entry (commonly referred to as 'certificates') required by the informant. The registrar then issues and certifies these for the informant.

A form is also issued on behalf of the Department for Work and Pensions (DWP) to assist the informant in dealing with state pensions, benefits and so on.

The registrar enters details of the registration onto the DWP's 'Tell-Us-Once' secure database if the informant wishes to use it. This gives the informant a unique reference number, which enables them to have many government-related concerns adjusted, such as council tax and electoral roll.[4]

Finally, the registrar issues a green form, which enables the funeral directors and crematorium or cemetery to proceed with the funeral. This form has a tear-off slip that must be returned to the registration office by the relevant party once the funeral has taken place. It is the registrar's responsibility to keep track of these slips to ensure that a legal burial or cremation has occurred.

How Did COVID-19 Change Things?

Prior to COVID-19, and the implementation of the Coronavirus Act the informant would be required to attend a registration office in person, having collected the MCCD from the relevant general practice (GP) or hospital, which they would then present to the registrar at their appointment. The exception to this would be in cases where a Coroner's post-mortem had taken place, in which case the Coroner's office would (and still do) issue an electronic form 100B (replacing the MCCD) direct to the registration office.

The registrar would have to carry out all the checks while the informant waited. The appointment time would be 30 minutes so any problems with the MCCD at that stage could result in delayed or wasted appointments.

Delays in actually booking appointments were also quite common, particularly in rural areas with a high elderly population such as Norfolk, where the informant might struggle to access transport to take them to the registration office.

As all the post-registration paperwork was issued to the informant, the funeral director, crematorium or cemetery would have to wait until the informant handed the green form to the funeral director in person. This could sometimes result in delays.

Following the implementation of emergency COVID-19 legislation registration appointments were permitted to take place via telephone, with the MCCD being electronically scanned and securely emailed over to the registration office prior to the appointment. The hard copy was then sent in the post. This meant that the registrar often has some time in which to check the MCCD's acceptability prior to the appointment. They could ring the surgery or hospital to chase the MCCD if it hadn't arrived, check acceptability of the causes of death or obtain information the doctor may have missed off. In some cases, a death can now be referred to the Coroner's office on a form 52 before the appointment time. Since the expiry of the Coronavirus Act 2020 legislation face to face registration is once again required.

The introduction of Medical Examiners (MEs) to the hospitals has saved registrars' time and brought them peace of mind. In some registration districts, MEs initial and date MCCDs, indicating that the MCCD has been completed after full ME scrutiny. It is ultimately a registrar's responsibility to be satisfied that the causes of death are acceptable, and they must carry out all statutory checks in all cases. However, knowing that an ME has been involved helps speed up the process. Where doubts still linger, MEs are usually forthcoming in allaying any fears. This also often means that the registrar will not have to contact the Coroner's office with these concerns. It is hoped that the introduction of MEs to the community will greatly reduce the need to question causes of death and other possible areas of uncertainty prior to registration.

During the COVID-19 emergency legislation if everything had been checked and found to be in order, the registrar could then telephone the informant at the appointment time, question them to obtain the appropriate information regarding the deceased, as before. Instead of signing, the registrar entered the informant's full name in the appropriate space on the registration, with the words 'information given by telephone' after it.

Certificate payment could be taken electronically and all documents posted to the informant with the exception of the green form, which would be scanned and securely emailed by the registration staff to the funeral director and crematorium or cemetery. This meant that the process of the funeral can be started immediately. Since the expiry of the Coronavirus Act on 25 March 2022 easements payments at registration for as many death certificates as are required can be made in person by card and thereafter more can be ordered online or by phone

Many informants reported that they found the experience of registering a death over the telephone a lot less stressful than having to come into the office to do so andit meant that registrations took place within the required five days more often and the process of funerals was expedited. It also meant that informants could register the deaths of loved ones from anywhere. A registration must be made in the district in which the death took place. Prior to the COVID-19 easements telephone registration meant that informants would have had to have come into the registration office in person or gone to their local office to register by 'declaration' which meant that all the paperwork would have to be sent to the 'in-district' registration office for registration, resulting in further delays.

The reversion to face-to-face registration following expiry of the Coronavirus Act 2020 has meant that some of the benefits of remote registration have been lost. However, the scanning and emailing of MCCDs to registration offices prior to appointments and the scanning and emailing of green forms from registration offices to crematoria, cemeteries and funeral directors has been retained and has greatly expedited the death registration and funeral process.

Conclusions

Registrars in England and Wales are statutory officers and all registrations have to be conducted in strict line with the Births and Deaths Registration Act (1953) and the Registration of Births and Deaths Regulations 1987. For a death registration from an MCCD issued by a doctor, this means within a timescale of five days where possible and in a manner that also allows for compassionate engagement with the relatives of the deceased.

Wrongly completed or late-arriving MCCDs waste time for registration staff and can also result in delays to appointments, distress to relatives and frustration to funeral directors, crematoria and cemetery management. It is hoped that the extension of the Medical Examiner Service to cover all deaths and the publication of this book will greatly reduce such issues in the future.

The introduction of the MEs to the hospitals has reduced the registrar's burden because it has meant that they do not have to contact the Coroner's office as frequently or worry about the contents of an MCCD. It is hoped that the wider introduction of this service will make the process of registering deaths faster and more efficient, to the benefit of all.

REFERENCES

1. Genealogy Archives. Births, Deaths, and Marriages Act, 1836. https://ukga.org/index.php?pageid=33382 (accessed 20 December 2021).
2. GOV.uk. Births and Deaths Registration Act, 1953. https://www.legislation.gov.uk/ukpga/Eliz2/1-2/20/data.pdf (accessed 20 December 2021).
3. The Royal College of Pathologists. Cause of Death List, 2020. https://www.rcpath.org/uploads/assets/c16ae453-6c63-47ff-8c45fd2c56521ab9/G199-Cause-of-death-list.pdf (accessed 20 December 2021).
4. GOV.uk. Department of Work & Pensions. Tell Us Once, 2021. https://www.gov.uk/after-a-death/organisations-you-need-to-contact-and-tell-us-once (accessed 20 December 2021).

CHAPTER 10

Role of the Coroner

Paul Marks

Introduction

Until 2013, Coroners operated under the Coroners Act 1988,[1] which was essentially a consolidation of the Coroners Act 1887[2]; Victorian legislation, in other words. At least two attempts had been made to reform the coronial jurisdiction in the twentieth century. The Wright Committee of 1936[3] recommended merging small coronial jurisdictions, and the Brodrick Committee,[4] which was formed in 1965 and reported in 1971, suggested some quite radical reforms, but both reports were largely disregarded.

A two-pronged stimulus for reform occurred at the turn of the millennium, one predicable, the other unexpected.

Tom Luce, always described as a senior civil servant, was tasked by the Home Office with chairing a fundamental review of the Coroner and death certification systems, and this reported in June 2003.[5] It concluded that neither the certification nor the investigation system was fit for purpose in modern society, and that substantial reform was needed.

The criminal activity of serial killer, Harold Shipman, a general practitioner who was found guilty of 15 counts of murder at Preston Crown Court in 2000, provided the unexpected drive to reform the coroners service and ensure that *all* deaths, whether suspicious or not, should be subject to scrutiny. There is evidence that Shipman probably killed somewhere in the region of 250 of his patients.

Dame Janet Smith, a High Court judge who chaired the Shipman Inquiry, reported her phase 1 findings in June 2002, which addressed the number of patients that were killed, and her phase 2 findings, which looked at death certification, cremation and the coroner, reported in July 2003.[6] Her findings were similar, but not congruent with those of Tom Luce, who subsequently took the differences into consideration, and published a position paper in 2004.[7]

The Fundamental Review and the Shipman Inquiry provided the necessary impetus for reform that culminated in the Coroners and Justice Act 2009,[8] but even then, it took until 25 July 2013 for the legislation to come into force and its form was diluted in comparison to its original provisions. Importantly, one of Dame Janet Smith's recommendations was to establish a Medical Examiner System to provide independent statutory scrutiny of *all* deaths. Indeed, sections 18–21 of the Coroners and Justice Act 2009 lay down the framework for such a service, which also provides for the appointment of a National Medical Examiner, a post currently held by Dr Alan Fletcher.

The organisation and operational aspects of the Medical Examiner Service are covered in detail in other chapters of this book, but this chapter will outline the important elements of the Coroner service, what coroners are and what they are not, and how the coroners' work interdigitates with the work of Medical Examiners. Coronial law is a complex subject and only an overview can be given in a chapter of this size, so interested readers are referred to standard texts in the further reading section.

Historical Development of the Coroner System

The ancient office of Coroner dates from the time of Richard I and was established through the Articles of Eyre in 1194. This provided for three knights and one clerk to 'keep the pleas of the crown' in each county. In Latin this was termed '*custos placitorum coronae*', which was corrupted to 'crowner' and then coroner. The duties of the mediaeval Coroner were more extensive and varied than his modern counterpart but essentially involved activities that raised revenue for the Crown. Coroners were known as *Crowners*, from which it is obvious how the current term derived. The office of Coroner remains the oldest judicial office in English law.

Some of the more unusual duties of the medieval Coroner are shown in Table 10.1, but it should be noted that whilst most have long since disappeared, coroners still have jurisdiction over treasure and operate under the provisions of the Treasure Act 1996.[9]

Up until July 2013, the Coroner service was based on the Coroners' Rules 1984[10] and the Coroners' Act 1988,[1] itself a consolidation of what, in essence, remained Victorian law. On 25 July 2013, the Coroners and Justice Act 2009[8] came into force and brought with it the Coroners (Inquests) Rules 2013[11] as well as other regulations (see below).

Table 10.1 Medieval Coroner's duties

- ☐ Tax collector – 'amercements'
- ☐ Investigation of sudden death
- ☐ Jurisdiction over felons
- ☐ The right of sanctuary
- ☐ Abduration of the Realm
- ☐ Trial by ordeal
- ☐ Treasure trove

Coroners and Justice Act 2009

The Coroners and Justice Act 2009 (the Act) received Royal Assent on
12 November 2009; however, it did not come into force until 25 July 2013.

At a number of points, it appeared that the Act would not come into force and
the office of Chief Coroner would not be filled. However, in September 2012, His
Honour Judge Peter Thornton QC became the first Chief Coroner of England
and Wales and has been responsible for the implementation of the Act and for
its accompanying rules and regulations. HHJ Mark Lucraft held office as Chief
Coroner until his preferment as Recorder of London and since 24 December 2020,
the office has been held by HHJ Thomas Teague, QC. There are two Deputy Chief
Coroners, one a judge and the other a senior coroner.

A number of provisions that had been incorporated into the original legislation
have not in fact materialised, including appeals of conclusions being heard by the
Chief Coroner.

One of the most significant changes introduced by the Act is the concept of the
investigation, which is distinguished from the *inquest* (see below).

The new Act also brought with it a change in terminology. Coroners' districts are
now referred to as coroners' areas; the Coroner in an area now becomes a *senior
coroner*. In the transitional arrangements between the old and new Acts, all deputy
coroners and all assistant deputy coroners become *assistant coroners* but in the new
hierarchy, a new post has been created, the *area coroner*. This is a full-time position and not every area has one. Area coroners tend to be appointed in the larger
and more complex coronial areas.

The Inquisition Form is now termed the *Record of Inquest* and the term 'verdict'
has been replaced by *conclusion as to the death*.

The Work and Organisation of the Coroner Service

The coroner's court is an inferior court of record (as opposed to a superior court
such as the High Court or Court of Appeal; inferior courts are subject to the
supervisory jurisdiction of the High Court) and is one of the few examples in
English law of an *inquisitorial* system, as opposed to an *adversarial* system.

A Coroner is an independent judicial officer who is appointed and paid by
the relevant local authority, but the appointment must be approved by the
Lord Chancellor and Chief Coroner. Once appointed, a Coroner can only be
removed from office by the Lord Chancellor with agreement of the Lord Chief
Justice.

There are currently 88 Coroner areas in England and Wales, and leadership and direction is provided by the Chief Coroner, who is a judge appointed by the Lord Chief Justice following consultation with the Lord Chancellor. The Chief Coroner is based at the Royal Courts of Justice and is supported by his or her own team and office.

To be appointed to coronial office, a prospective applicant must satisfy the *judicial eligibility criteria,* be under the age of 70 years and receive approval for appointment from the Lord Chancellor and Chief Coroner. Legally qualified medical practitioners cannot be appointed to office unless they are also solicitors, barristers or Fellows of the Chartered Institute of Legal Executives, thereby fulfilling the judicial eligibility criteria. A popular misconception, based on confusion with the use of the term the USA (and other countries) is that coroners are forensic pathologists.

The situation in Northern Ireland is slightly different as there is a unified coroners service governed by the Department of Justice and headed by a High Court judge.

Investigation

One of the most significant changes that the 2009 Act has brought in, is the concept of the *investigation* and this is detailed in section 1 of the Act. A consequence of the investigation is that a Coroner will no longer need to open an inquest to release a body for funeral purposes.

The duty to investigate pursuant to section 1 is:

(1) A senior Coroner who is made aware of the deceased person is in that coroner's area must as soon as practicable conduct an investigation into the person's death if subsection (2) applies.
(2) This subsection applies if the Coroner has reason to suspect that:
    (a) the deceased died a violent or unnatural death,
    (b) the cause of death is unknown, or
    (c) the deceased died while in custody or otherwise in state detention.

Interestingly, a Coroner is able to conduct preliminary inquiries under the authority of section 1(7) of the Act and this seeks to determine whether section 1(1) is engaged. Such inquiries would typically comprise a post-mortem examination. The Act does not define post-mortem examination and this is deliberate, to permit alternatives to invasive post mortem such as CT or MRI scanning to be employed.

If a natural cause of death is found as a result of the post-mortem examination, then the Coroner is obliged to discontinue the investigation and inform the next of kin or personal representatives of this in writing.

If the cause of death is natural but has occurred in state detention or custody, the Coroner must in these circumstances continue to investigate and proceed to inquest.

Referral of Deaths to the Coroner

Deaths are notified to the Coroner in the circumstances shown in Table 10.2.

A statutory requirement for such reporting is the responsibility of the Registrar of Births and Deaths (Regulation 41 of Registration of Births and Deaths Regulations 1987) but in practice, the Coroner will take referrals from a large number of sources including medical practitioners, Medical Examiners, family members, police and funeral directors.

Following referral, the Coroner will decide whether to investigate the case further. It may be that following discussion with the relevant doctor, sufficient information is available to permit a natural cause of death to be recorded and subsequently registered. In these circumstances, the Coroner can issue a certificate known as *Form 100A* that enables the Registrar of Births, Deaths and Marriages to register the death without a post-mortem examination. This form supports the certificate of the medical cause of death issued by the doctor.

If, however, the cause of death is unknown, the Coroner will order a post-mortem examination and if the cause is *natural,* can issue *Form 100B,* which permits the death to be registered following the post-mortem but without recourse to inquest.

There is little doubt that the routine work of a coroner's office, culminating in the disposal of cases by issuing Form 100A and 100B, will represent, at least in numerical terms, the majority of the caseload. However, the high-profile work, which in terms of cases is far less, are inquests. In approximate terms, for every ten referrals, only one inquest will need to be opened and concluded.

Table 10.2 Circumstances when deaths are notified to the Coroner

- No doctor saw the deceased during his or her last illness
- Whilst a doctor may have attended the deceased during the last illness, the doctor is not able or available, for any reason, to certify the death
- The cause of death is unknown
- The death occurred during an operation or before recovery from the effects of an anaesthetic
- Death occurred at work or was due to industrial disease or poisoning
- The death was sudden and unexplained
- The death was unnatural
- Death was due to violence or neglect
- The death was in other suspicious circumstances, e.g. suspected suicide
- Death may be due to an abortion
- Death occurred in prison, police custody or another type of state detention
- All deaths of children and young people under 18, even if due to natural causes. This is for safeguarding purposes
- Death may be linked to an accident, *however long ago it happened*

The Legal Basis for Ordering a Post-Mortem Examination

Coroners operate under the Coroners and Justice Act 2009 (the Act) and their powers in relation to post-mortem examinations and power to remove a body are set down in Sections 14 and 15 respectively. Readers are referred to these sections of the Act as well as to the Chief Coroner's Guidance No 32,[12] which covers post-mortem examinations including second post-mortem examinations.

The important points raised in this guidance are: *'Whilst a Coroner has legal control over the body of a deceased person, it is for the Coroner to decide whether to commission a first or subsequent post-mortem examination and it is for the Coroner to decide whether to permit a second examination of the body on the instruction of an interested party. Despite there being a widespread misconception (particularly in homicide cases), there is no automatic right to a second post-mortem examination and requests should be scrutinised rigorously by the Coroner on a case-to-case basis.'*

What Is a Post-Mortem Examination?

The Act does not define what constitutes a post-mortem examination; this is not an omission but is deliberate so that methods other than invasive post mortem, where appropriate, can be employed to determine the cause of death. These would include CT or MRI scanning, limited post-mortem examination, toxicology alone and external examination only, to name but a few.

Adjournment

After receiving evidence of identification of the deceased, the Coroner will open and adjourn the inquest to a date and time to be set down pending further investigation. In homicide cases, the inquest will typically not be resumed, as the matters a Coroner needs to address will inevitably be ventilated in the Crown court. An exception to this would be if there was a murder/suicide, in which case both inquests would need to be resumed and concluded.

Inquests

In the above section the distinction between an investigation and an inquest has been made, but in what circumstances will an inquest need to be held?

Section 1(2) and s4(2) of the Act require that an inquest is held where a Coroner is made aware that the body of a person is within his or her area and that there is reason to suspect that:

- The deceased has died a violent or unnatural death
- The cause of death is unknown
- The deceased died whilst in custody or otherwise in state detention.

The remit of an inquest is limited and set out in s5 of the Act but on occasions, a Coroner may have to sensitively but firmly manage expectations. An inquest is required to address four limited but factual questions, which are:

(a) Who the deceased was
(b) How, when and where the deceased came by his or her death
(c) The particulars (if any) required by the 1953 Act to be registered concerning the death.

Section 5(3) of the Act prohibits the senior Coroner or the jury from expressing any opinion on any other matter and s10(2) prohibits any *determination* being framed in such a ways as to appear to determine any question of:

(a) Criminal liability on the part of a named person, or
(b) Civil liability.

In the majority of cases in which an inquest is held, the Coroner will sit alone. Indeed, s7(1) of the Act requires a Coroner to sit alone unless the requirements in s7(2) are fulfilled. Under these certain circumstances, it is incumbent on them to sit with a jury, but s7(3) provides a discretionary power to sit with a jury empaneled.

Approximately 3% of inquests are heard with a jury that comprises between 7 and 11 jurors who are randomly selected from the electoral role.

Section 7(2) of the Act provides that:

An inquest into a death must be held with a jury if the senior Coroner has reason to suspect:

(a) That the deceased died while in custody or otherwise in state detention, and that either:
    (i) The death was a violent or unnatural one
    (ii) The cause of death is unknown
(b) That the death resulted from an act or omission of:
    (i) a police officer
    (ii) a member of a service police force in the purported execution of the officer's or member's duty as such, or
(c) that the death was caused by a notifiable accident, poisoning or disease.

During jury cases, as a point of procedure, if advocates address the Coroner on points of law or make submissions, these are heard in the absence of the jury. The task of the jury is more complex in coronial cases than it is in criminal cases, where it is a matter of deciding guilt or otherwise.

After all the evidence is adduced in a jury case, the Coroner must sum up the case and direct the jury as to the relevant law and leave them with conclusions to consider. He or she must draw the jury's attention to sections 5(1) and 5(3) of the Act, as well as the prohibitions in respect of civil and criminal liability as stated in s10(2).

Types of Inquest

The vast majority of inquests are 'common law', ordinary or 'Jamieson inquests'. This would best be described as a 'standard inquest', where the wider circumstances surrounding the death are not explored. However, the European Convention on Human Rights,[13] as enshrined in our domestic law by the Human Rights Act 1998,[14] in particular Article 2, provides that everyone's life shall be protected by law. This has important ramifications and consequences for inquests in which Article 2 is engaged, where deaths might have involved *agents of the state.*

Article 2 provides for two substantive duties and an implied obligation. The state has a negative duty to refrain from taking life and a positive duty to protect life by setting up an appropriate infrastructure of laws and practices to ensure this. It also means that there is an implied procedural obligation to investigate deaths by an effective and independent public body in which it might be arguable that the state has breached its negative or positive obligations. In these circumstances an 'enhanced' or 'Middleton inquest' will occur. Instances where such a hearing would be set down might include prison deaths, police shootings and deaths of detained psychiatric patients. In physically ill patients who die in hospital, in certain circumstances, Article 2 might be engaged but this would be determined on a case-by-case basis.

An enhanced inquest will permit the Coroner or jury to go into further detail and in practical terms, this means that the question *how* the deceased came by his or her death is expanded to include *by what means and in what circumstances* the deceased met his or her death.

It should be noted that at present legal aid is generally not available for most inquests but it can be made available for inquests in which Article 2 is engaged.

Standard of Proof

The standard of proof required in a coroner's court is the *civil* standard of proof – on the balance of probabilities, whether an event is more likely to have occurred than not, or if expressed mathematically, a 51/49% split in the evidence. This now applies to *all* coroner's conclusions, formerly known as verdicts. Prior to the UK Supreme Court handing down judgement in the case of R (Maughan) v HM Senior Coroner for Oxfordshire [2020] UKSC46,[15] suicide and unlawful killing were determined to the criminal standard of proof, *beyond reasonable doubt.*

Evidence

The rules of evidence are not as strict in the coronial jurisdiction as in other jurisdictions. For example, *hearsay* evidence is admissible. Evidence in a coroner's court comes in two basic forms: evidence heard on oath in the witness stand pursuant to rule 20 (1) of the Coroners (Inquests) Rules 2013; and documentary evidence. Rule 23 of the Coroners (Inquests) Rules 2013 permits written evidence to be admitted in the absence of the person who has made the statement. There are however a number of conditions and safeguards that must be addressed before such evidence can be used. The Coroner must be satisfied that:

(i) it is not possible for the maker of the written evidence to give evidence at the inquest hearing at all, or within a reasonable time;

(ii) there is good and sufficient reason why the maker of the written evidence should not attend the inquest hearing

(iii) there is good and sufficient reason to believe that the maker of the written evidence will not attend the inquest hearing; or

(iv) the written evidence (including evidence in admission form) is unlikely to be disputed.

It is important to note that *before* such evidence is admitted under this authority, the Coroner must announce in open court the nature of the evidence, the full name of the author, and that interested persons may object to such admission and their entitlement to seeing a copy of the evidence.

Before the Inquest

In particularly complex or contentious inquests, a *pre-inquest review hearing* (PIR) may be held. Prior to the 2009 Act, PIRs were held and acknowledged to be good practice for case management, but rule 6 of the Coroners (Inquests) Rules 2013 has put them on a formal basis. An agenda should be provided to all interested persons and a PIR will address matters such as the scope of the inquest, whether Article 2 ECHR is engaged, whether a jury is required, the need for independent expert evidence, what evidence will be heard and what will be dealt with under rule 23, who are designated as *interested persons,* together with other matters such as the date and duration of the final hearing.

Disclosure

The 2009 Act brought with it a far wider duty to disclose reports and documents. The presumption now is for *full* disclosure to take place to *interested persons* (see below), but there is limited discretion under rule 15 of Coroners (Inquests) Rules 2013 to refuse a request for disclosure, if that request is unreasonable.

Interested Persons

An interested person is not someone who has some idle curiosity about the case, but someone defined as such within s47(2) of the Act. Such persons would include relatives, personal representatives of the deceased, a beneficiary under a policy of insurance or insurance company, a trade union representative, a person who may have by his actions or omissions caused or contributed to the death, a person appointed by, or representative of, an enforcing authority, a chief constable and so on. The Coroner has a discretion to accord interested person status, if he or she thinks that individual has a sufficient interest.

The significance of being an interested person is essentially twofold. Firstly, it entitles the interested person to disclosure and secondly, it allows the interested person to examine a witness either directly or through an advocate.

Witnesses at inquests are generally compellable and refusal to attend without proper reason is a contempt of court. Coroners are well aware of attempts by witnesses not to attend court by presenting a 'sick note', but inability to attend work needs to be carefully distinguished from being unfit to attend court.

A statutory protection exists for witnesses against *self-incrimination* under rule 22 of the Coroners (Inquests) Rules 2013. This means that a witness is not obliged to answer if he or she has been asked an incriminating question. In such circumstances, the Coroner must inform the witness that they are not obliged to answer. Of course, a witness may choose to waive this right and answer if they wish. As the term *incriminate* would suggest, the privilege only extends to criminal proceedings and not to civil or disciplinary proceedings.

Conclusions

Conclusions are in general of two types, *short form* and *narrative.* The Chief Coroner has issued guidance about short form and narrative conclusions. The outcome of an inquest is set out in the *Record of Inquest* and will show the medical cause of death and the conclusion, short form or narrative.

The Coroner or jury, having heard the evidence and decided upon the medical cause of death, need to arrive at the conclusion by a three-stage process, namely:

- Make findings of fact based upon the evidence.
- Distil from the findings of fact *how* the deceased came by his or her death.
- Record the conclusion, which must be consistent with the other stages.

The Chief Coroner advises that wherever possible, short form conclusions should be returned. These might include accidental death, misadventure, suicide, drugs/

alcohol, natural causes, unlawful killing, lawful killing, open, road traffic collision, industrial disease and so on.

Narrative conclusions are becoming increasingly common, and some argue that this may be due to the widening of circumstances in which they can be employed due to Article 2 of ECHR. The case law relating to this is highly specialised, but interested readers are directed to the further reading section for guidance on this.

A narrative conclusion must not offend against (breach) s5(1) or s10(2) of the Act, but acts or omissions may be recorded. For example, during the procedure, the common bile duct was inadvertently transected or a 'T' tube was not left in the common bile duct. However, expressions suggestive of civil liability such as 'carelessness' or 'neglect' should be avoided.

An example of a narrative conclusion that does not identify an individual or offend against s5(1) and S10(2) might be: *'The deceased was admitted for elective resection of a colonic carcinoma but in the post-operative period developed an anastomotic leak, which was not recognised for five days, during which time appropriate investigations and treatment were not undertaken. He subsequently died from peritonitis and multi-organ failure. An opportunity existed to diagnose and treat this anastomotic leak and if taken, the deceased would not have died on 1 February 2009.'*

In short form conclusions, if the facts support a conclusion that an opportunity to treat a patient was missed and that such treatment, on the balance of probabilities, if administered would have resulted in survival, then the Coroner can add the rider of *neglect*. For example, a surgical operation may have gone wrong, and the post-operative management was woefully inadequate. If the evidence adduced shows that the deceased's condition was known, or should have been known as such, for action to have been taken, and that this omission amounted to gross failure and that there was a clear and causal relationship with the death, then a conclusion of *misadventure to which neglect contributed* may be recorded. The test, as set out in Lord Bingham's judgement in R v HM Coroner for North Humberside ex parte Jamieson,[16] is stringent and a high bar to jump.

Aftermath

On concluding an inquest, a number of administrative matters need attention, notably issuing the *Record of Inquest* and supplying the Registrar of Deaths with a form 99 (certificate after inquest).

Although the Act initially made provision for appeals to be made to the Chief Coroner in respect of inquest conclusions, this had not occurred, and the relevant legislation was repealed during debates on the Public Bodies Bill 2011.[17]

There are two remedies whereby the conclusion of a coroner's court can be examined by the High Court. The first is by *judicial review* and the second is by the statutory remedy pursuant to s13 of the 1988 Coroners Act, which remains in force.

Judicial review is a complex area of law and is quite distinct from an appeal where there is a rehearing of the case by a superior court. With judicial review, consideration is given to process and, for example, whether the procedure was unreasonable, unfair or failed to take into consideration relevant evidence. The process is time limited to three months for the submission of an application.

A section 13 fiat brought under the 1988 Act is not time limited, however, and confers upon the High Court certain powers, but these can only be exercised with the authority of the Attorney General.

Typical reasons for an application include refusal to hold an inquest, an inquest being unsatisfactory due to insufficiency of inquiry, rejection of relevant evidence, fraud or irregularity of proceedings or, importantly, where new facts or evidence have emerged.

The High Court can order that an inquest is held or quash the original Record of Inquest, and a new hearing occurs.

Prevention of Future Deaths

Under the1988 Coroners Act and the Coroners Rules 1984, there was provision for a Coroner to make a report under the authority of rule 43 to prevent future deaths and this represented an important public health and safety measure. Although the rule was 'strengthened' in 2008, it still lacked 'teeth'.

Coroners now have a *duty* to report under regulation 28 of the Coroners (Investigations) Regulations 2013.[18]

Such *reports to prevent future deaths* can now be made at an early stage without needing to await the conclusion of the inquest. However, the Coroner is required to have considered all the documents, evidence and information that are relevant before making the report. This regulation imposes a duty upon the Coroner to report the matter to a person whom the Coroner believes may have power to take action.

A *response* pursuant to Regulation 28 must contain details of any action taken or that is proposed to be taken or an explanation as to why no action is proposed. The response must be provided within 56 days.

Relationship with Medical Examiners

Clearly, the roles of Coroner and Medical Examiner are different but there is some overlap, and it is vital that coroners have a good working relationship with their Medical Examiner colleagues. Indeed, the Chief Coroner in Guidance No. 31[19] emphasises the importance of this and states at paragraph 13:

'It is the firm view of the Chief Coroner that coroners (and in particular, senior coroners) should forge good collaborative working relationships with Medical Examiners in their area in much the same way as they have with Registrars. Medical Examiners are now part of the wider death oversight and investigation system in England and Wales. Their duties are different to coroners but they are the counterpart for coroners and coroners and their staff should work in a spirit of partnership and mutual respect with the Medical Examiner.'

Coroners should ensure that there is a direct line of communication between themselves and the Medical Examiners, and they are encouraged to sit on the appointment committees for Medical Examiners. This helps to foster good relations and most importantly serves to place the bereaved at the centre of the process.

REFERENCES

1. Coroners Act 1988. https://www.legislation.gov.uk/ukpga/1988/13/contents (accessed 28 January 2022).
2. Coroners Act 1887. https://www.legislation.gov.uk/ukpga/Vict/50-51/71/contents/enacted (accessed 28 January 2022).
3. Wright RAW. Committee on Coroners. (Cmbd 5070) HMSO 1936.
4. Brodrick Committee. Report of the Committee on Death Certification and Coroners (Cmnd 4810). HMS0, November 1971.
5. Luce T. Death Certification and Investigation in England, Wales and Northern Ireland: The Report of a Fundamental Review 2003 (Cmnd 5831).
6. Smith J. The Shipman Inquiry. Third Report. Third Report. Death Certification and the Investigation of Deaths by Coroners (Cmnd 5854) 2003. https://assets.publishing.service.gov.uk/government/uploads/system/uploads/attachment_data/file/273227/5854.pdf (accessed 28 January 2022).
7. Luce T. Death Certification and the Coroner Service. Medicine, Science and the Law 2004 44 4 287–289 https://doi.org/10.1258/rsmmsl.44.4.287 (accessed 7 February 2022).
8. Coroners and Justice Act 2009. https://www.legislation.gov.uk/ukpga/2009/25/contents (accessed 28 January 2022).
9. Treasure Act 1996. https://www.legislation.gov.uk/ukpga/1996/24/contents (accessed 28 January 2022).
10. Coroners Rules 1984. https://www.legislation.gov.uk/uksi/1984/552/contents/made (accessed 28 January 2022).
11. The Coroners (Inquests) Rules 2013. https://www.legislation.gov.uk/uksi/2013/1616/contents/made (accessed 28 January 2022).

12. Chief Coroner. Guidance No. 32 Post-Mortem Examinations including Second Post-Mortem Examinations. 2019. https://www.judiciary.uk/wp-content/uploads/2019/09/Guidance-No.-32-Post-Mortem-Examinations-including-Second-Post-Mortem-Examinations.pdf (accessed 28 January 2022).
13. European Convention on Human Rights. https://www.echr.coe.int/Documents/Convention_ENG.pdf (accessed 28 January 2022).
14. Human Rights Act 1998. https://www.legislation.gov.uk/ukpga/1998/42/schedule/1 (accessed 28 January 2022).
15. R (on the application of Maughan) (AP) (Appellant) v Her Majesty's Senior Coroner for Oxfordshire (Respondent). UKSC 2019/0137. https://www.supremecourt.uk/cases/uksc-2019-0137.html (accessed 28 January 2022).
16. R v North Humberside and Scunthorpe Coroner ex parte Jamieson: CA 27 Apr 1994.
17. Public Bodies Act 2011. https://www.legislation.gov.uk/ukpga/2011/24/contents (accessed 28 January 2022).
18. The Coroners (Investigations) Regulations 2013. https://www.legislation.gov.uk/uksi/2013/1629/contents/made (accessed 28 January 2022).
19. Chief Coroner. Guidance No. 31 Death Referrals and Medical Examiners. 2019. https://www.judiciary.uk/wp-content/uploads/2019/09/Guidance-No.-31-Death-Referrals-and-Medical-Examiners.pdf (accessed 28 January 2022).
20. The Coroners Allowances, Fees and Expenses Regulations 2013. https://www.legislation.gov.uk/uksi/2013/1615/contents/made (accessed 28 January 2022).

CHAPTER 11

The Medical Examiner Service: Relationship with Mortality Governance

Berenice Lopez

Background

Concern about deaths due to problems in care, patient safety and scrutiny of mortality has intensified in the UK over recent years with the extensive coverage of investigations into National Health Service (NHS) care failures.[1-5] This has informed two major policy initiatives – the National Learning from Deaths (LfD) programme[6] and the Medical Examiner system.[7]

The National Learning from Deaths guidance was developed in response to failures at Southern Health NHS Foundation Trust[4] and subsequent highlighting, by the regulator of healthcare in England (the Care Quality Commission), of poor systems across the NHS for organisational LfD. The report concluded that LfD was not being given sufficient priority in some NHS organisations and valuable opportunities for improvements were being missed.[8] It clearly identified the need for organisations to engage with bereaved families and carers and to recognise their insights as a vital source of information. The CQC now requires all NHS trusts to 'say something about every death'.

In March 2017, NHS England launched the Learning from Deaths (LfD) initiative. Evidence-based approaches for mortality reviews were combined with a mechanism for strengthening transparency and governance to create this framework. The LfD guidance recommends that NHS trusts employ systematic case sampling and retrospective case record review (RCRR) by a recognised methodology to review deaths, identify remedial safety problems and address them with an emphasis on engagement and disclosure with bereaved families and carers. The guidance provides the minimum requirements for selecting cases for RCRR. These are based on those most likely to yield opportunities for learning and improvement, including deaths where bereaved families and carers or staff have raised a significant concern about the quality and safety of care. No specific methodology for RCRR was stipulated but the structured judgement review (SJR) methodology, as used in the National Mortality Case Record Review programme,[9] was recommended.

DOI: 10.1201/9781003188759-11

To support the need for transparency and accountability, every trust is required to publish a policy for how it responds to, and learns from, deaths under its care, including its approach to case record review. Trusts are also required to publish data on the total number of deaths, those subject to review, and those judged more likely than not to have been due to problems in care (as ascertained by RCRR) alongside a summary of key learning, improvement activities and challenges relating to LfD both internally and externally (trust quality accounts). The requirement to publish data on potentially preventable deaths has proved controversial not least because numbers of these deaths are low, judgements on preventability are often very difficult and the public disclosure of this data conflicts with the desired focus on learning.[10] Community and mental health NHS trusts are also required to have their own LfD policy.

The guidance also recognises the specific, recognised processes and programmes that focus on the deaths of children,[11] people with learning disabilities,[12] maternal deaths and stillbirths[13] and mental health homicides (independent investigation). These are covered by other approaches and governance arrangements but are also important sources of learning from deaths.

Since it was first published in 2017, LfD guidance has been extended to ambulance trusts,[14] specific guidance has been published on working with families[15] and work continues to improve systems for learning from the deaths of children and people with learning disability. However, a means of ensuring all deaths are scrutinised independently has been missing, as has a means by which the input of bereaved families and carers is assured for every death. These are being provided by the Medical Examiner initiative.

Introduction of Medical Examiners

The introduction of Medical Examiners (MEs) responds to a number of inquiries, including the Shipman Inquiry's conclusions, which highlighted the need for greater scrutiny of deaths not reported to the Coroner (and hence better safeguards to the public). MEs have also been recommended by other independent inquiries into failings in the NHS as a means of identifying avoidable deaths and problems in care[2,3] (see Chapter 1). The passage of the Coroners and Justice Act 2009[16] provides the legal basis for this new role, but it is not yet a statutory requirement. The requirement for input from bereaved relatives is a unique aspect of the ME approach. In addition, interaction with front-line clinical staff may provide information on system level issues not recorded in the patient's case notes. Some of these elements may be delegated to an appropriately qualified Medical Examiner Officer (MEO). Standards for the delivery of Medical Examiner Services (MES) have been published by the Medical Examiners Committee of the Royal College of Pathologists.[17] The national roll-out of the ME system commenced in April 2019.

By serving as the initial filter for all deaths, referring those with potential problems in care for RCRR, the ME system can be seen as naturally complementary to the

LfD initiative, offering a single, robust framework for mortality review. The jury is still out, however, on how these processes actually work alongside each other and there are no published data to support ME screening of deaths to inform the selection of cases for RCRR, although this is awaited.[18]

Nonetheless, these initiatives together have the potential to foster openness, transparency, improved engagement with bereaved families and carers, and broader surveillance of clinical care for improvement. However, they both also need to reconcile the potentially competing goals of encouraging learning with the need for accountability. There is a clear overlap between the LfD requirement to identify and report deaths more likely to be due to problems in care and the ME services' role in deterring criminal activity and identifying poor practice. Beyond scrutiny of case notes, MEs may need to speak to staff and check records of safety incidents. Staff may find this difficult if this is not handled sensitively as they may feel challenged in their practice and or professionalism.

In recognition that most care delivery problems belong to the system, and in recognition of the futility of blame,[19] it is vital that the right balance is struck and these initiatives align to create a receptive milieu for the continued development of a culture of reflection, learning and improvement that delivers psychological safety for staff. This does not preclude accountability for the rare cases of reckless or neglectful care or indeed, for organisations to put LfD into practice.

MEs will interface with all mortality review processes, not simply the LfD programme. The National Medical Examiner (NME) has produced guidance on how MEs and MEOs should interact when reviewing the deaths of patients with learning disabilities and/or autism (LeDeR) with bereaved families and carers, colleagues including LeDeR colleagues, and partners.[20] Further clarification will be required on how the ME system will interact with other mortality review processes and programmes such as those that focus on the deaths of children, maternal deaths and stillbirths.

Independence of Medical Examiners

Credibility and flexibility

A key principle of the MES is independence of scrutiny. Medical Examiners must be able to review deaths objectively and impartially, without fear or favour, away from local political considerations and criticism and without being assumed to have an agenda beyond fulfilling the duties of their role. It is the practical ways that this principle is given effect that may impact on political and public perceptions of the services' credibility.

The twin issues of independence and credibility raise questions about the set-up of the MES – can ME offices be hosted by NHS providers whose patients' deaths are being scrutinised and still claim to be independent? Can NHS consultants employed by acute providers be appointed to Medical Examiner posts within that organisation? Who selects the MEs – the organisation or an outside body? The affiliations and experience of the MEs also strongly affects credibility.

A balance between credibility and flexibility has had to be struck, at least for now. Currently, ME offices are hosted by acute hospital sites in England, and MEs are not required to be independent of the organisation whose patients' deaths are being scrutinised. MEs in Wales are employed by NHS Wales Shared Services Partnership and therefore have a greater degree of independence from their main employer. General practitioners (GPs) are already an integral part of many ME services, having been recruited into the role of ME before the MES extends to cover community deaths.

Medical Examiners are accountable to the NME via the structure outlined in Chapter 2. However, there is also a line of accountability to the NHS organisation that employs them. It is important for host organisations to manage and have oversight of the performance of the ME service including timeliness of review, referrals for RCRR and other internal governance systems, unusual patterns and trends of concerns and the impact of the service on linked processes such as timeliness of MCCD completion and Coroner's referrals. The organisation also needs to have sight of any complaints about the service from relatives or staff as well as Coroner or registry office concerns. ME scrutiny of deaths will generally fall under existing mortality governance and/or bereavement and mortuary managerial arrangements in host organisations with a reporting line to an appropriate oversight committee, typically the organisation's LfD committee. There is an inherent tension between protecting independence and ensuring accountability.

The relationship between MEs with host organisations and the Regional Medical Examiner in England has been clarified in good practice guidelines by the National Medical Examiner.[21] This states that the management and oversight of Medical Examiners rests with local line management arrangements with the responsible employer. A strong commitment from an organisation's leadership is an important factor in facilitating independence of review. However, MEs have recourse to the Regional Medical Examiner in England or the Lead Medical Examiner for Wales if they are not satisfied that concerns they have raised about the quality and safety of care have been resolved by the organisation or that influence is being exercised over their independent role. There is also clear advice for MEs on the types of cases where their independence may be questioned, for example the death of a patient they or their department cared for or where they are professionally or personally related to someone who provided care or are personally related to the deceased. It should be hoped that all MEs will recognise these actual or perceived conflicts.

Professional accountability to the General Medical Council is perceived to help safeguard the independence of the MEs. Furthermore, it could be argued that MEs' sense of independence and accountability instilled as part of training are at least of equal importance and must be emphasised. Structural protections are still important but may need to be considered in terms of their impact on MEs' exercise of courage and integrity.

Independence and interdependence

Another grey area is how the MES can interface with their organisation's own mortality and wider safety governance arrangements in terms of people, processes and systems. The NME states that MEs should build on existing services and take local practice into account. However, MEs also need to align with the national model and will be part of a distinct system with its own funding arrangements.[21]

On a practical level, ME offices need to work with local administrative and clinical governance teams to access paper-based patient case notes where these are used and ensure concerns about quality and safety of care are notified. Given the multiple internal clinical governance routes within a hospital system, MEs may need to seek guidance as to which route is most appropriate for a specific case. ME offices may be expected to report patient safety incidents via the organisation's risk management system, refer cases to the organisation's RCRR process or escalate cases to the serious incident process where appropriate, report a safeguarding concern and/or inform a quality improvement report (QIR) for concerns relating to care provided by external organisations. Some cases may need to be referred for clinical review at specialty mortality and morbidity meetings. MEs may also need to refer bereaved families and carers to patient experience services such as the Patient Advice and Liaison Service (PALS).

It is also important for MEs to be able to obtain feedback on their notifications and referrals, particularly as many MEs highlight a lack of meaningful feedback as limiting scope for development.[22] For example, information on what learning has been captured from an RCRR, from cases referred or reviewed but not referred by the ME and what changes have been made as a result, may help to inform future reviews and ensure consistency of referrals. How such feedback is obtained may vary depending on local set-up but could involve communication with staff in corporate risk, patient safety and other clinical governance teams. The interaction cannot be a one-way process. For example, the organisation's mortality lead may find it helpful to ask the MES to pay particular attention to particular types of cases, for example deaths in a specific diagnosis group or procedure that have triggered a mortality outlier alert. The mortality lead may also need to have sight of the outcome of previous ME reviews as part of the initial investigation into this alert.

Allowing for both sides of the equation encourages collaboration, and helps to bring everyone into alignment with each other and invested in the same goals.

A number of trusts have electronic mortality review and analysis systems that capture ME, 'parent team' mortality and morbidity reviews and RCRRs providing a complete record of reviews for patients who have died, preserving institutional knowledge and providing an integrated LfD solution. Important advantages are the elimination of the information governance, confidentiality and legibility issues associated with paper and the provision of a robust audit trail. Information needed to assess an MES can also be captured readily. Access to completed RCRR and associated reviews on these systems may help individual MEs follow up their referrals. Data access controls, however, must clearly be robust, and may be one of the most challenging parts of the relationship between LfD and the MES.

Use of an electronic ME template, aligned to national recommendations, can help ensure a common approach to scrutiny and, by means of compulsory fields, completeness of record. This may also facilitate the collation of ME insights across reviews over time to support the timely identification of trends and patterns of concern within an organisation or, as the service expands to the non-acute sector, across a wider healthcare system. Given that most MEs do not concurrently cover a service and have limited opportunity for formal team contact,[22] such a system is potentially very valuable. These issues may become more problematic as the service rolls out to the community, the number of MEs and MEOs within an office increases and care quality concerns are notified to a wider array of NHS and non-NHS providers. In addition, both MEs' and other mortality reviewers' insights can be collated across all reviews and triangulated with other sources of mortality intelligence supporting organisations and the wider system to understand where to focus improvement work.

Nationally, there are plans to introduce a 'digital product to capture scrutiny' to support the ME system.[23] This will be hosted by the NHS Business Services Authority, which will provide service support and ongoing development. As yet it appears to be a stand-alone product to be used exclusively by the ME system with no clarity as to its inter-operability with local platforms or accessibility outside the MES. Whilst this approach provides further structural protection of MEs' independence and a mechanism by which scrutiny data can be collected at a national level, the risks associated with digital silo working need to be taken into consideration. Such risks include the potential for additional complexity, duplication and more work, as well as communication problems. This approach could also be viewed as going against a desirable focus on localism in the delivery of improvement projects.[24]

Quality of Care, Patient Safety and the Medical Examiner

Whilst the ME service enables organisations to meet the CQC requirement to 'say something about every death', it is not yet clear just how reliably the service identifies safety concerns or its overall impact on improving patient safety and quality of care.

A review of over 23 000 deaths scrutinised by ME pilot sites in Sheffield and Gloucester, funded by the Department of Health and Social Care in 2016, reported improved referrals to the Coroner, improved accuracy of MCCD completion and that input from bereaved relatives was assured. It also found ME review of deaths was a consistent source of high quality information about quality of care, irrespective of the nature of the problem and irrespective of the type of organisation involved.[25] Analysis of ME reviews in one of the pilot services identified clinical governance concerns in 4% of cases that attending doctors were unaware of.[25] The most recent NME report, based on formal submissions from ME offices in England and Wales for the period January to December 2021, included vignettes demonstrating the positive impact of the ME service on patient safety and the experience of bereaved families and carers. Data published in this report suggest that MEs are referring 10% of deaths scrutinised for RCRR or other clinical governance process because of concerns about care.[23] These data thus far lend credence to the potential valuable role of this service in improving patient safety, but clearly there is much more to be done.[26]

Important learning could, however, be missed if ME assessment is too limited or the threshold for notification to clinical governance including referrals for RCRR is set too high. The National Institute for Health Research Policy Research Programme has funded a study involving ME pilot sites that will compare the findings of ME assessment and RCRR by structured judgement review (SJR). This will provide useful information on how these processes work together and will determine how ME screening influences the workload and yield of information from SJR. Results are awaited.[18]

There is already evidence of variation within and between ME services around how they address potential care quality problems. This may relate to differences in the perceived salience of information sources, most notably information received from relatives, and implicit criteria for referral decisions. These in turn, may be linked to individual and service preferences as well as different organisational pathways for referral of care quality concerns.[22] Protected time for training and support, team contact and robust mechanisms for feedback have been suggested to address reviewer variation.[8,22]

In the interim, despite the lack of data, some host organisations have, pragmatically, replaced previous mortality screening approaches based on 'parent team' reviews of all deaths in their care with the ME review to avoid duplication and to free up clinical staff who are already carrying out mortality and morbidity reviews, RCRRs, Coroner s' reports, incident investigations, complaint responses and clinical audits, often on the same cases. Additional random sampling of cases for RCRR, from all those reviewed by the MES but not referred to RCRR or other governance systems, can provide insight into whether the local service's thresholds for referral are appropriate. The outcome of these reviews can be fed back to the service for shared learning and to help improve consistency. These RCRRs may also be used to provide a rich source of learning from care that goes well, in the form of everyday clinical work, supporting Safety-II approaches to learning and improvement.[27] The RCRR methodology supports this but, all too often, the assumption is made that learning only comes from care that goes wrong.

Deaths More Likely Due to Problems in Care

The RCRR methodology can also be used to make a judgement about whether a death was potentially avoidable. Studies using RCRR in NHS hospitals in England have estimated that up to 5.2% of deaths were probably avoidable.[28–30] Judging avoidability of death, however, is a complex assessment that can be challenging to undertake. This is because assessment goes beyond judging quality and safety of care by also taking into account such issues as comorbidities and estimated life expectancy. The evidence indicates that levels of agreement can be very low when assessing potential avoidability of death. Large samples with multiple reviewers would be needed to ensure reliability rendering this impractical and expensive. The original NMCRR SJR template included an avoidability scale but there was a subsequent move away from attempting to judge avoidability by the Royal College of Physicians, NHS Improvement and other national bodies. The preferred language used is 'deaths being more likely than not due to problems in care'. However, a reframe does not make this judgement any easier to make. In addition, room for improvement in the quality of care is more common than preventability of death, thus undue focus on preventability may lead to missed opportunities for learning, particularly where death was more likely to be expected. The validity and utility of identifying deaths due to problems in care through RCRR remains questionable, although this can inform decisions to escalate specific deaths to an organisation's serious incident process and trigger an organisation-wide or system-wide response. These deaths can also act as a powerful lever for improvement.

It is worth noting that ME scrutiny is intended to identify care quality concerns requiring further investigation. It is not intended to determine preventability. In addition, there is evidence of missed opportunities for learning if the ME focus is exclusively on identifying issues implicated in the cause of death.[22] Quality of care rather than avoidable mortality should be the focus, not least because of the importance of assessing the quality of care provided to patients at the end of life.

Learning from Deaths in Community Settings

There is a long history of using deaths as comparative, benchmarking measures for performance monitoring of patient safety in acute NHS care settings. The examination of deaths to drive learning and improvement in quality of care is also well established in acute care settings; at a local level with mortality and morbidity (M&M) meetings, clinical audits, case record reviews, investigation of incidents and mortality outlier alerts, and at a national level via clinical databases, run by various bodies including professional societies, which assess in-hospital and 30-day mortality, confidential enquiries and the output of the NHS National Reporting and Learning System. Systems of mortality surveillance and review are not, however, well established in primary care. In addition, whilst acute, community, mental health and ambulance trusts are required to implement an LfD policy, there is, at present, no such requirement for primary care.

Routine monitoring of general practice mortality was recommended by the Baker report following the Shipman murders.[31] However, this recommendation has proved challenging for a number of reasons.[32] These include the need for high quality mortality data linked to general practices,[33] complexities in case-mix adjustment,[34] problems identifying special cause from random variation[35,36] and an agreed process for following up concerns. To date, no national approach to benchmarking mortality in primary care has been implemented.

Patient safety in primary care has also not been explored to the same extent as in the hospital setting. International evidence suggests that the error rate is around 2–3% of primary care consultations and that around 4% of these incidents may be associated with severe harm including death. Incidents relating to diagnosis and prescribing were most likely to result in severe harm.[37] Despite these figures, only a small proportion of the patient safety incidents reported to the NHS National Reporting Learning System come from primary care. Whilst work is being done to improve reporting by improving access and feedback, the roll-out of the MES to primary care will provide an additional structure for insight in this setting.[38] In addition, improving patient safety often involves addressing the issues that occur when patients move between primary and secondary care. The MES will be well placed to provide insight into patient safety threats relating to care pathways spanning these and other care settings.

A key question is how primary care will respond to notifications from the MES in the absence of an established framework for LfD. The framework may need to evolve from existing approaches to learning and reflection such as significant event analysis. Another key issue, given that many patient safety issues arise at care transitions reflecting the quality of the interaction between primary and secondary care, is how these issues are notified to providers and investigated. A limitation of the RCRR is its focus on the quality and safety of care provided during a patient's final admission (or indeed to care provided up to and including discharge) with no flexibility to include pre-hospital care or care provided during a previous hospital admission. Of note, the National Quality Board is currently reviewing LFD guidance. It may be that any future iteration of this guidance will consider a system-wide approach to mortality governance which takes into account the need for whole pathway approaches to mortality review and the need for a system-wide approach to mortality governance by the new NHS integrated care systems.

ME review of deaths in the community could be seen as the 'raison d'être' for the service and long overdue given that it was originally recommended in response to deaths in this setting. However, the complexities of this aspect of the roll-out have been recognised and advice to proceed slowly and carefully is wise.[39] Of note, the ME pilot sites were mainly based in hospital care so extending the system to primary care may well uncover additional and potentially unforeseen problems.

Conclusions

The LfD and ME systems should contribute substantially to patient safety, care and learning. The integration of these systems whilst maintaining the independence and integrity of the ME role has many challenges. A pragmatic approach drawing on the most effective elements of review of deaths in acute hospitals and the community should ensure that the intended benefits of both systems are maximised.

REFERENCES

1. Dame Janet Smith. The Shipman Inquiry, Third Report: Death Certification and the Investigation of Deaths by Coroners, 2003. https://www.gov.uk/government/uploads/system/uploads/attachment_data/file/273227/5854.pdf (accessed 21 December 2021).
2. Francis R. Report of the Mid-Staffordshire NHS Foundation Trust Public Inquiry, 2013. https://www.gov.uk/government/publications/report-of-the-mid-staffordshire-nhs-foundation-trust-public-inquiry (accessed 21 December 2021).
3. Kirkup B. The Report of the Morecambe Bay Investigation, 2015. https://assets.publishing.service.gov.uk/government/uploads/system/uploads/attachment_data/file/408480/47487_MBI_Accessible_v0.1.pdf (accessed 21 December 2021).
4. NHS England. Independent Review of Deaths of People with a Learning Disability or Mental Health Problem in Contact with Southern Health NHS Foundation Trust, 2015. https://www.england.nhs.uk/south/wp-content/uploads/sites/6/2015/12/mazars-er-rep.pdf (accessed 21 December 2021).
5. Gosport Independent Panel. Gosport War Memorial Hospital. The Report of the Gosport Independent Panel, 2018. https://www.gosportpanel.independent.gov.uk/media/documents/070618_CCS207_CCS03183220761_Gosport_Inquiry_Whole_Document.pdf (accessed 21 December 2021).
6. National Quality Board. National Guidance on Learning from Deaths. https://www.england.nhs.uk/wp-content/uploads/2017/03/nqb-national-guidance-learning-from-deaths.pdf (accessed 21 December 2021).
7. NHS England. The National Medical Examiner System. https://improvement.nhs.uk/resources/establishing-medical-examiner-system-nhs/ (accessed 21 December 2021).
8. Care Quality Commission. Learning, Candour and Accountability. A review of the way NHS trusts review and investigate the deaths of patients in England, 2016. https://www.cqc.org.uk/sites/default/files/20161213-learning-candour-accountability-full-report.pdf (accessed 21 December 2021).
9. Royal College of Physicians. National Mortality Case Record Review Programme, 2019. https://www.rcplondon.ac.uk/projects/national-mortality-case-record-review-programme (accessed 21 December 2021).
10. Lalani M, Hogan H. A narrative account of the key drivers in the development of the Learning from Deaths policy. *J Health Serv Res Policy*. 2021; 26: 263–271.

11. GOV.uk. Department of Health and Social Care for Education. Child Death Review: Statutory and Operational Guidance (England), 2018. https://assets.publishing.service.gov.uk/govern ment/uploads/system/uploads/attachment_data/file/859302/child-death-review-statutory-and-operational-guidance-england.pdf (accessed 21 December 2021).

12. NHS England and NHS Improvement. Learning from Lives and Deaths: People with Learning Disability, 2017. http://leder.nhs.uk (accessed 21 December 2021).

13. University of Oxford. MBRRACE-UK: Mothers and Babies: Reducing Risk through Audits and Confidential Enquiries across the UK, 2021. https://www.npeu.ox.ac.uk/mbrrace-uk (accessed 21 December 2021).

14. National Quality Board. National Guidance for Ambulance Trusts on Learning from Deaths: A framework for NHS ambulance trusts in England on identifying, reporting, reviewing and learning from deaths in care, 2019. https://www.england.nhs.uk/wp-content/uploads/2019/07/learning-from-deaths-guidance-for-ambulance-trusts.pdf (accessed 21 December 2021).

15. National Quality Board. Learning from Deaths: Guidance for NHS trusts on working with bereaved families, 2018. https://www.england.nhs.uk/wp-content/uploads/2018/08/learning-from-deaths-working-with-families-v2.pdf (accessed 21 December 2021).

16. GOV.uk. Coroners and Justice Act 2009, 2009. http://www.legislation.gov.uk/ukpga/2009/25/contents (accessed 21 December 2021).

17. Royal College of Pathologists. Standards for the Delivery of the Medical Examiner Service. https://www.rcpath.org/uploads/assets/ba3248d6-ec8b-4179-a635e3ceabe1fda6/Medical-Examiners-Provisional-Standards-for-Service-Delivery.pdf (accessed 21 December 2021).

18. National Institute for Health Research. Evaluation of Medical Examiners' Review to Identify Potentially Avoidable Deaths due to Problems in Care, 2017. https://fundingawards.nihr.ac.uk/award/PR-R16-0516-23001 (accessed 21 December 2021).

19. National Advisory Group on the Safety of Patients in England. A Promise to Learn – A Commitment to Act. Improving the Safety of Patients in England, 2013. https://assets.publishing.service.gov.uk/government/uploads/system/uploads/attachment_data/file/226703/Berwick_Report.pdf (accessed 21 December 2021).

20. NHS England and NHS Improvement. Implementing the Medical Examiner System: National Medical Examiner's Good Practice Guidelines, 2020. https://www.england.nhs.uk/wp-content/uploads/2020/08/National_Medical_Examiner_-_good_practice_guidelines.pdf (accessed 21 December 2021).

21. The Royal College of Pathologists. National Medical Examiner's Good Practice Series No. 3. Learning Disabilities and Autism, 2021. https://www.rcpath.org/uploads/assets/daf86eaa-d591-40d5-99d54118d10444d2/Good-Practice-Series-Learning-disability-and-autism-For-Publication.pdf (accessed 21 December 2021).

22. O'Hara R, Coster J, Goodacre S. Qualitative exploration of the Medical Examiner role in identifying problems with the quality of patient care. BMJ Open. 2021; 11: e048007.

23. NHS England and NHS Improvement. National Medical Examiner's Report 2021. https://www.england.nhs.uk/publication/national-medical-examiner-reports/ (accessed 5 July 2022).

24. Collins B. Fenney D. Improving Patient Safety through Collaboration. A Rapid Review of the Academic Health Science Network Patient Safety Collaboration, 2019. https://www.ahsn network.com/app/uploads/2019/03/Improving-patient-safety-through-collaboration.pdf (accessed 21 December 2021).

25. Furness PN, Fletcher AK, Shepherd NA, et al. Reforming Death Certification: Introducing Scrutiny by Medical Examiners. Lessons from the pilots of the reforms set out in the Coroners and Justice Act 2009, 2016. https://assets.publishing.service.gov.uk/government/uploads/system/uploads/attachment_data/file/521226/Death_certificate_reforms_pilots_-_report_A.pdf (accessed 21 December 2021).

26. Fletcher A, Coster J, Goodacre S. Impact of the new medical examiner role on patient safety. *BMJ*. 2018: 363; k5166.
27. Hollnagel E, Wears RL, Braithwaite. From Safety–I to Safety–II: A White Paper, 2015. https://www.england.nhs.uk/signuptosafety/wp-content/uploads/sites/16/2015/10/safety-1-safety-2-whte-papr.pdf (accessed 21 December 2021).
28. Hogan H, Healey F, Neale G, et al. Preventable deaths due to problems in care in English acute hospitals: a retrospective case record review study. *BMJ Qual Saf.* 2012; 21: 737–745.
29. Hogan H, Zipfel R, Neuburger J, et al. Avoidability of hospital deaths and association with hospital-wide mortality ratios: retrospective case record review and regression analysis. *BMJ*. 2015; 351: h3239.
30. Roberts AP, Morrow G, Walkley M, et al. From research to practice: results of 7300 mortality retrospective case record reviews in four acute hospitals in the North-East of England. *BMJ Open Qual.* 2017; 6: e000123.
31. Baker R. Harold Shipman's Clinical Practice 1974–1998: A Clinical Audit Commissioned by the Chief Medical Officer. London: The Stationery Office; 2001.
32. Baker R, Jones D, Goldblatt P. Monitoring mortality rates in general practice after Shipman. *BMJ*. 2003; 326: 274–276.
33. Bhopal R. Fallout from the Shipman case. Death registers in general practice would be a means of preventing malpractice and murder [letter]. *BMJ*. 2000; 320: 1272.
34. Mohammed A, Booth K, Marshall D. A practical method for monitoring general practice mortality in the UK: findings from a pilot study in a health board of Northern Ireland. *BJGP*. 2005; 55: 670–676.
35. Frankel S, Sterne J, Smith GD. Mortality variations as a measure of general practice performance: implications of the Shipman case. *BMJ*. 2000; 320: 489.
36. Pinder DC. Monitoring the death rates of general practitioners' patients in a single Health Authority. *J Public Health Med* 2002; 24: 230–231.
37. Panesar SS, deSilva D, Carson-Stevens A, et al. How safe is primary care? A systematic review. *BMJ Qual Saf.* 2016; 25: 544–553.
38. NHS England and NHS Improvement. The NHS Patient Safety Strategy: Safety Culture, Safety System, Safer Patients, 2019. https://www.england.nhs.uk/wp-content/uploads/2020/08/190708_Patient_Safety_Strategy_for_website_v4.pdf (accessed 21 December 2021).
39. NHS England and NHS Improvement. Extending Medical Examiner Scrutiny to Non-acute Settings, 2021. https://www.england.nhs.uk/wp-content/uploads/2021/06/B0477-extending-medical-examiner-scrutiny-to-non-acute-settings.pdf (accessed 21 December 2021).

CHAPTER 12

The Medical Examiner Service in the Community

Katie Ann Carpenter

Introduction

The Medical Examiner (ME) system in England and Wales has developed as part of a series of reforms to the system of death certification. Weaknesses in this system were first identified over 20 years ago in Dame Janet Smith's inquiry[1] into the murders committed by English general practitioner Dr Harold Shipman. Convicted in January 2000 on the basis of 15 test cases, it is likely Shipman killed at least 200 other patients in the community. Such cases are fortunately very rare, but an effective ME system clearly needs to be implemented in the community setting as soon as possible to provide appropriate safeguards.

For understandable reasons, the non-statutory ME system introduced in 2019 has focused largely on acute hospital deaths to date. It has always been clear, however, that the next implementation phase would be to include deaths in all other settings. The coronavirus pandemic has obviously led to delays, but work is now in progress to make this aspiration the reality. The commitment to a statutory ME system in the Health and Care Act 2022 highlights the need for rapid development of the ME Service in the community.[2] This is vital – there are approximately 550 000 deaths in a typical year in England and Wales, and about 50% of these occur outside acute hospitals.[3] National Medical Examiner Dr Alan Fletcher emphasised the importance of the community setting in the Fourth Annual Leeming lecture,[4] reminding all we must *'mind the gap'* and continue to develop our services to develop an inclusive approach to deaths wherever they occur.

Alongside the release of a suite of resources on the FutureNHS Collaboration Platform,[5] a letter confirming this next phase of implementation was sent to all primary and secondary care providers on 8 June 2021.[6] ME offices are now moving towards scrutinising deaths in people's own homes, as well as a range of other settings including care homes (nursing and residential), community hospitals and hospices (NHS and independent). They should also include non-coronial deaths of patients being cared for by mental health trusts and independent healthcare providers. Deaths within prisons would be outside the remit of the ME service as these would all be routinely notified to the Coroner.

As well as the Welsh community experience described in Chapter 2, some of the early ME service pilots in England also included community deaths. The first pilot began in Sheffield in 2008 and included a third of its general practices.[7] Although the six subsequent pilot schemes established with Department of Health funding were mainly focused on hospital deaths, a few did consider community cases.[8] These pilots demonstrated *'numerous clear benefits'*[9] and are valuable implementation resources, which will have informed the guidance[5] recently published by the National Medical Examiner team. Writing in 2018, National Medical Examiner Dr Alan Fletcher was realistic that *'extending the system to primary care is likely to involve additional and potentially unforeseen problems'*[10] so teams will inevitably need to take a proactive, flexible approach.

This chapter considers the challenges ME offices in England face as they begin to widen their scrutiny to include community deaths. It is important to note that ME implementation in Wales included the community setting from 2020, and their approach is described separately in Chapter 2. By reviewing the three mandatory steps of scrutiny first, and then considering other key principles all ME offices must uphold (as highlighted in the National Medical Examiner's good practice guidelines),[11] the particular challenges of community extension are considered. Approaches to implementation across England are then discussed and relevant process issues highlighted.

Three Components of Scrutiny

There are three mandatory steps involved in the ME scrutiny process. These are now reviewed in turn, giving the opportunity to consider the challenges of each when extending services to cover non-acute deaths. Having this awareness at the outset will support ME offices in England when starting to implement within community settings.

Medical record review

The medical record review is the first key aspect of scrutiny and requires MEs to have sight of the relevant case notes. With offices based in acute hospitals, accessing the notes of patients dying within these is usually a straightforward process. Accessing the relevant clinical records of patients dying in community settings presents more of a challenge, however, and therefore needs early consideration when planning the roll-out.

Encouragingly, the early community pilots in Sheffield and Gloucester suggested *'obtaining notes from primary care did not cause significant problems or delays, because an adequate summary of most primary care notes could be obtained in electronic form'.*[8] In Gloucester, they were also able to access case records from an independent hospice electronically. Pilot site reviews did acknowledge occasional difficulties accessing records *'for patients who had moved practices or moved to a different hospital in the short period of time before their death'.*[8] It is important to recognise that when electronic records were unavailable at the pilot sites, they relied on faxed transmission of relevant paper documents. Since these pilots, fax machines have been banned within NHS organisations in favour of other communication methods (such as secure email) to improve patient safety and cyber security. This means ME offices must use alternative, secure approaches.

Once teams are clear which locality areas and care settings fall within their office remit, a key first step is thus to consider how MEs will access the relevant notes. The national team does not suggest a 'one size fits all' implementation model, and very much acknowledge that areas of England vary hugely in terms of geography, rurality and healthcare provision. It is also abundantly clear that the ideal of interoperability of IT systems does not match the reality in many areas. Resources for ME offices contained in the FutureNHS Collaboration Platform[5] include a range of approaches that might be used. A recent paper[12] describing one team's experience demonstrated how working closely with existing local electronic referral processes might provide a workable, practical solution.

General practitioner (GP) notes are all now electronic, but different practices use different health record systems (such as SystmOne and EMIS Health). ME offices will need to be able to have read-only access to all those systems in use in their area. Alternatively, they might choose to develop processes whereby GP practice staff can send them a summary record including a final entry from the treating doctor who will certify death (qualified attending practitioner [QAP]). If ME office staff are going to be accessing the records directly, they will obviously need the relevant access rights and training to do this. Teams need to ensure data protection laws are followed, given the sensitive nature of such data transfer.

Other healthcare providers such as hospices or mental health trusts may use different electronic or paper notes – discussions will be needed with each provider to find a solution for MEs being able to access the relevant case notes in a timely way. It is not realistic to think MEs will be able to review paper case notes away from their acute hospital base.

Data sharing between providers has been an ongoing concern with legal barriers and challenges that took time to resolve. Included within the resources on the FutureNHS Collaboration Platform[5] are some legal documents to reassure teams and providers. These include a 'Data Sharing Statement' summarising the approved application[13] under Regulation 5 of the Health Service (Control of Patient Information) Regulations 2002 ('section 251 support') to process confidential information without consent. There is also a template 'Organisational Assurance Statement for Medical Examiners' that offices can adapt to use within their NHS Trust. It is expected that these documents provide the required assurances such that local data sharing arrangements will not be needed.

Qualified attending practitioner discussions

The second essential component of the scrutiny process is discussion with the QAP. The aim of this is to review the proposed cause of death and determine whether the Coroner needs to be notified. When ME offices are reviewing cases in the non-acute setting, they therefore need to set up efficient processes of liaising with QAPs in a range of different locations, often working variable and different shifts. Using an electronic ME-1A form or equivalent as recommended in the national good practice guidelines[11] gives offices the opportunity to request helpful information from these doctors. For example, the Norfolk and Norwich University Hospital ME office template includes core data fields requesting contact details and availability for the QAP (as well as those for any alternative doctors) to avoid delays and minimise difficulties contacting them. The example processes set out in Annex A and B of the letter sent to all providers on 8 June 2021,[6] and reinforced by documents on the FutureNHS Collaboration Platform,[5] make clear these interactions can be completed by correspondence (e.g. email) and a verbal discussion is not normally required. As with scrutiny of acute deaths, all discussions with the QAP must be clearly documented within the MES data management system.

Talking to the bereaved

The final key component to ME scrutiny is asking the bereaved whether they have questions about the cause of death, or concerns about the care their loved one has received. This must be done in a compassionate way and ME Services (MES) need to be able to respond to concerns raised. The importance and relevance of these discussions is the same irrespective of place of death. Of note, the early community pilots identified cases where significant safety concerns were detected through this scrutiny process. A review highlighted one occasion when notification of information from two different families concerning care concerns in a nursing home led to a Coroner's investigation.[8] These next of kin discussions make a real difference, and are just as important for patients dying in non-acute settings. As public awareness of the ME role increases so families will be better prepared for these calls. There is helpful public awareness information on the FutureNHS Collaboration Platform[5] that teams can use to support this.

Other Key Principles Underpinning Medical Examiner Office Functions

The National Medical Examiner's good practice guidelines[11] detail key principles, in addition to the three components of scrutiny already discussed, that must always be upheld. These are equally relevant for community ME Services, and hence these principles are now reviewed in turn to allow consideration of the impact of each for the roll-out.

Partnership working

As services start to expand their working into community settings, so collaboration and close working with all stakeholders will be paramount. Such working fits with the legislative proposals for a Health and Care Bill set out within the February 2021 White Paper.[2] There is no doubt that the coronavirus pandemic has been one of the greatest challenges our health service has ever experienced. Nonetheless it has led to amazing examples of integration, new ways of working and a pace of change unimaginable previously. The White Paper proposes that *'different professions, organisations, services and sectors will work with common purpose and in partnership'*[2] (p.7). Whilst there is no doubt extending Medical Examiner services to non-acute settings will be a challenge, it may be that the time is right for barriers to be more easily overcome.

The National Medical Examiner team have been liaising with relevant partners in the lead up to the community roll out. These include the Independent Healthcare Providers Network, the Royal College of General Practitioners and the British Medical Association as well as representatives from national faith groups. As Medical Examiner services start to roll out to the community, they too will then need to focus on partnership working involving all relevant stakeholders. Within the FutureNHS Collaboration Platform resources[5] is a 'Checklist and Information for Local Stakeholder Engagement', which is an excellent starting point for teams. Table 12.1 identifies these stakeholders.

In order to work effectively with all these partner organisations, there is a need for good communication and engagement at both national and local levels (Table 12.1). The National Medical Examiner office already has good lines of communication and processes in place. Locally, teams need to build on this to ensure the many different stakeholders understand the changes resulting from the ME system. Offices will need to develop the processes necessary to be able to provide a full service by April 2023. Local information campaigns, targeting both the public and professional stakeholders, are helpful and important[14] but will have to be funded from within the existing budget. There has been largely positive engagement with stakeholders in the initial phase of MES work in acute hospitals and the creation of local implementation groups. It may well be more difficult engaging with community partners, particularly in the context of an ongoing pandemic and vaccination programme. Primary and secondary care are equal partners in this important work, and it is very important this is clear from the outset. Although hosted by secondary care, ME Services are independent and must ensure primary care colleagues do not feel they are being 'inspected' or 'criticised' by hospital colleagues. Having general practitioners (GPs) working as MEs will help mitigate this

Table 12.1   Stakeholders and considerations required for community ME scrutiny

Patient groups and the bereaved	These must be at the heart of the process and teams will need to empower and consult in their local areas.
Healthcare providers	Outside the acute hospital setting, there is a range of other places where patients may die. ME Services (MES) need to link with providers of healthcare in all these settings. These might include care homes (nursing and residential), community hospitals, hospices (NHS and independent) and charitable or local authority care providers. There may also be small numbers of patients dying in beds run by mental health trusts and independent healthcare providers. It is important to remember that MES are based in acute hospital trusts and also need to liaise with their own organisation. A business case will likely be needed to ensure they are aware of the direction of travel in terms of service development and to support the necessary recruitment. Office space and equipment availability is an important factor and must be planned for at an early stage with host trusts. Service level agreements may need setting up with other trusts.
Coroner's office	These working relationships will already be in place with the acute NHS trust MES, but interactions will obviously increase as the scope of deaths being reviewed by ME teams increases. Some offices may need to move to engaging with more than one Coroner's office. The 2019 Notification of Deaths Regulations and associated guidance[15] has helped clarify those cases doctors need to refer to the Coroner, and will hopefully minimise local variations in practice, although many doctors are unaware of the new regulations.
Registration services	As with Coroners, ME offices will already be working in partnership with their local teams. The recent Royal College of Pathologists Cause of Death List[16] will have helped clarify common areas of difficulty. Registration services will need to be reassured that introduction of community Medical Examiner services will not lead to increased numbers of five-day breaches.
NHS staff	Including mortuary and bereavement services, PALS, doctors, nursing staff, allied health professionals, governance and patient safety teams. Again, these relationships will likely already be established but ongoing liaison will be vital as services begin to undertake community scrutiny.
Neighbouring Medical Examiner Services	Close collaboration and 'sharing experiences and expertise to support learning'[11] is important and will also help minimise potential difficulties in boundary areas. In Norfolk with three ME Services, different IT systems are used to record scrutiny. It is intended that the three services share an electronic ME1A form and process. This means that the local community NHS trust will only have to follow one process for deaths in all their community hospitals.
Other stakeholders	These will vary from area to area but will likely include local faith groups, funeral directors, cremation and burial services and Healthwatch.

risk. ME teams can use the range of resources on the FutureNHS Collaboration Platform[5] to inform their communication and engagement work.

Establishing credibility – delivering a timely, efficient and effective service

To maintain the credibility and independence of this new system as it extends to cover community deaths, MEs and MEOs '*should demonstrate the highest professional standards at all* times'.[11] To do this, every effort must be made to deliver timely, efficient and effective services. Most ME Services have a target of completing scrutiny within 24 hours of the case records notes being available. Table 12.2 identifies specific challenges and operational requirements that need to be considered in developing community Medical Examiner services in regards to these key principles of timeliness, efficiency and effectiveness.

Table 12.2 Specific challenges and operational requirements regarding consideration when developing community Medical Examiner Services to support the key principles of timeliness, efficiency and effectiveness

Notification of deaths	In developing community models, the starting point needs to be developing effective processes to notify ME offices of deaths. The provision of records to the office is discussed earlier in the chapter.
Availability and prioritisation	To provide a timely MES within the community, offices must be open at times '*that meet the needs of the local population, with cover for staff on leave*'.[11] Teams need to consider the need and nature of out-of-hours provision, based on the religious and other needs of the local population. Recent guidance from the National Medical Examiner's Good Practice Series (No 2) covers urgent release of a body and includes deaths within the community.[17] Joint working with neighbouring ME offices might enable sharing of duties such as out-of-hours cover.
Non-forensic examination of bodies	This was always going to be a challenge in developing timely community ME models. Pilots found such examinations were only necessary in a small proportion of cases,[8] and the logistics were challenging, particularly in rural and isolated areas.[14] Consequently, it was concluded that an external examination need not be mandatory and could be delegated to others.[8] The 2020 Coronavirus Act further changed practice within England and Wales such that this is no longer a routine requirement of the cremation process. Cremation Form 5 has not been re-introduced on expiry of the Coronavirus Act on 24 March 2022.
Delegation of tasks	As the volume of cases being scrutinised approximately doubles with extension to community deaths, it will be even more important that teams review their approach to this. For the system to be flexible and efficient, Medical Examiner Officers must be used effectively to '*enable Medical Examiners to focus on their role and to facilitate cost-effective operation of the Medical Examiner office*'.[11]
IT and data collection	This is a key challenge in the planning of community services. GPs and hospitals use different case management systems. As well as the logistical difficulties of accessing patient records already considered, teams must have effective IT systems to allow them to process cases and link to existing systems. In Wales, a single MES including the community has been established via four regional hub offices. Cases are recorded on a single digital system, which provides the required quarterly reporting for the National Medical Examiner and also provides '*analysis and reporting integrated with health board governance systems*'.[18] Implementation of an NHS Business Services Authority digital product to capture scrutiny across the Medical Examiner system, and a digitalised Medical Certificate of Cause of Death, is planned for April 2023, or when the statutory system begins.[11] Until then, teams will need to develop digital data collection systems that meet relevant requirements and fit local circumstances as they build community activity. Some aspects of data collation will be more challenging outside the acute setting. For example, unlike hospital cases, it will not be so easy to identify the outcome of coronial referral or the mechanism of disposal of the body. These are key data fields and may impact on funding of the service. In addition, teams will need to ensure their IT systems enable concerns and compliments to be raised with the relevant community providers.
Completing the process	Once the full ME scrutiny process has been completed, it is important that systems are in place to confirm that this is reflected within the final Medical Certificate of Cause of Death (MCCD). Some acute NHS trust teams in collaboration with registration offices use stamps on the MCCD to confirm they have been authorised for release by a ME. A different process will be needed for scrutiny within the community. The FutureNHS Collaboration Platform resources[5] suggest ME offices might issue case reference numbers in releasing the final MCCD so it is clear for registration services. This will become easier once the certificates are electronic.
Workforce issues	National Medical Examiner Dr Alan Fletcher recently identified workforce and training (via the Royal College of Pathologists) as one of the three pillars of the ME system.[4] Professionalism is clearly essential in terms of establishing credibility as a service developing within the community. Offices will need a diverse team (ideally including GPs) to help build links across the healthcare system and with communities. The coronavirus pandemic has understandably led to recruitment freezes and further delays might ensue if further waves occur, putting teams under potential pressure in the build-up to roll out of the statutory system. NHS staff are tired and need time to reflect and recover. This may impact on offices being able to recruit enough Medical Examiners and officers to upscale scrutiny numbers to include community deaths. The excellent availability of online training will support development of new staff. For professional development, it is important mechanisms are in place to facilitate direct team communication. A recent paper highlighted lack of structures for providing meaningful feedback and learning were '*particular areas of weakness in most of the ME services*'[19] they surveyed.

Escalating concerns

MES are required to escalate concerns about the care in individual cases as appropriate, to the Coroner or local clinical governance teams.[11] Escalation of clinical governance concerns in community cases is more difficult than in the acute setting. ME offices must be able to work with existing local clinical governance and mortality review processes across a range of providers, so an initial scoping exercise is key prior to roll-out. This may be best managed by a multi-disciplinary local implementation group. Services must establish clear links to ensure learning or feedback identified during the scrutiny process is shared with the care provider for consideration or review.

Independence

As with scrutiny of hospital cases, it is essential that independence is maintained. Offices must have processes in place to ensure MEs do not scrutinise cases where their independence may be questioned.[11] It is therefore important as offices plan their roll out into community, and work closely with other services to do this, they must always retain demonstrable independence.

Approaches to Implementation and Process Issues to Consider

In January 2020, the planned timeframe for the non-statutory system in regards to community scrutiny was set at 2020/21.[11] The pandemic has led to slippage of this timeline and ME Services are being actively encouraged to work with local partners to widen scrutiny to all non-coronial deaths within a specified geographical area. The National Medical Examiner is strongly advising ME offices to *'adopt an incremental approach to local implementation'*.[11] This means that until the statutory system is in place (April 2023 at the earliest), two approaches will be running in parallel as not all cases will go through the ME process. It makes sense for ME offices to focus initially on working with those stakeholders who are keen and able to engage.

In England, the Regional Medical Examiner offices are working closely with, and providing support for, local ME offices to plan for this next phase of scrutiny of community cases. ME offices have been provided with expected numbers of community deaths within their area and discussions are underway to ensure logical allocation of cases to each office. The aim in the East of England is to follow our Coroners' jurisdictions in terms of boundaries. Other areas are taking different approaches – London is allocating by boroughs, and others by local authority areas. Integrated Care Systems are at the heart of the legislative proposals for a new Health and Care Bill[2] and these will be increasingly key and relevant to implementation models.

Conclusions

It is very clear that the process of extending ME scrutiny to community settings is complex and will need careful planning and collaboration. In England and Wales, the coronavirus response saw collaboration within the health and care system accelerate at a pace and scale previously unimaginable. Whilst it is important the NHS has time to reflect and begin recovery from the pandemic, this collaboration needs to be utilised in this next phase of implementing ME scrutiny in the community. It is vital to get to a position where there is equal scrutiny irrespective of place of death.

To succeed in their community roll-out, ME office teams must be ambitious and adopt a joined-up approach based on collaborative relationships. They will need to work together and flexibly, making good use of technology whilst always keeping the patient at the heart of the process and remaining focused on the needs of the bereaved. There is no doubt that the extension of ME scrutiny to non-coronial deaths in community settings will be challenging. The benefits however will be significant, in terms of both contributing to improvements in patient care and providing assurance for the public. Further delays in implementation must be avoided – after all, it has already been over 20 years since Dr Harold Shipman was convicted.

REFERENCES

1. GOV.uk. The Shipman Inquiry, Third Report: Death Certification and the Investigation of Deaths by Coroners, 2003. https://www.gov.uk/government/uploads/system/uploads/attachment_data/file/273227/5854.pdf (accessed 20 December 2021).
2. Health and Care Act 2022. www.legislation.gov.uk/ukpga/2022/31/contents/enacted (accessed 13 6 2022).
3. Fletcher A. National Medical Examiner's Report 2020, 2021. https://www.england.nhs.uk/wp-content/uploads/2021/04/B0413_NME-Report-2020-FINAL.pdf (accessed 20 December 2021).
4. Fletcher A. The Fourth Annual Leeming Lecture. Centre for Contemporary Coronial Law, University of Bolton, 2021.
5. FutureNHS Collaboration Platform. https://future.nhs.uk/MedicalExaminerResources/grouphome (accessed 20 December 2021).
6. NHS England. System Letter: Extending Medical Examiner Scrutiny to Non-acute Settings, 2021. https://www.england.nhs.uk/publication/system-letter-extending-medical-examiner-scrutiny-to-non-acute-settings/ (accessed 20 December 2021).
7. NHS Improvement. Pilot of the Department of Health Medical Examiner, 2017. https://www.england.nhs.uk/wp-content/uploads/2021/07/Pilot-of-the-Department-of-Health-medical-examiner.pdf (accessed 20 December 2021).
8. GOV.uk. Reforming Death Certification: Introducing Scrutiny by Medical Examiners, 2016. https://assets.publishing.service.gov.uk/government/uploads/system/uploads/attachment_data/file/521226/Death_certificate_reforms_pilots_-_report_A.pdf (accessed 20 December 2021).
9. Ellis P. Medical Examiners and Death Certification Reform: Still in the Long Grass, 2019. https://docsbay.net/medical-examiners-and-death-certification-reform-still-in-the-long-grass (accessed 20 December 2021).

10. Fletcher F, Coster J, Goodacre S. Impact of New Medical Examiner Role on Patient Safety. *BMJ.* 2018; 363 (1–4): k5166.
11. NHS England. Implementing the Medical Examiner System: National Medical Examiner's Good Practice Guidelines, 2020. https://www.england.nhs.uk/establishing-medical-examiner-system-nhs/#national-medical-examiners-good-practice-guidelines (accessed 20 December 2021).
12. Sarkhel T, Richardson R, Lane J. Community roll-out of the Medical Examiner Service: electronic referral service. http://www.rcpath.org" www.rcpath.org. July 2022;199: 655–657.
13. NHS Health Research Authority. Confidentiality Advisory Group registers, 2021. https://www.hra.nhs.uk/planning-and-improving-research/application-summaries/confidentiality-advisory-group-registers/ (accessed 20 December 2021).
14. Local Government Association. Introduction of Medical Examiners and Reforms to Death Certification in England and Wales, 2017. https://www.local.gov.uk/parliament/briefings-and-responses/introduction-medical-examiners-and-reforms-death-certification (accessed 20 December 2021).
15. Ministry of Justice. Guidance for Registered Medical Practitioners on the Notification of Deaths Regulations, 2019. https://www.nottinghamcity.gov.uk/media/3372367/moj-guidance-for-registered-medical-practitioners-on-the-notification-of-deaths.pdf (accessed 20 December 2021).
16. The Royal College of Pathologists. Cause of Death List, 2020. https://www.rcpath.org/uploads/assets/c16ae453-6c63-47ff-8c45fd2c56521ab9/G199-Cause-of-death-list.pdf (accessed 20 December 2021).
17. The Royal College of Pathologists. National Medical Examiner's Good Practice Series No. 1, 2021. https://www.rcpath.org/uploads/assets/72675084-5ed3-43a1-b518c61395dd1194/Good-Practice-Series-BAME-paper.pdf (accessed 20 December 2021).
18. NHS England. National Medical Examiner Update, 2020. https://www.iccm-uk.com/iccm/wp-content/uploads/2020/12/December-2020-NME-bulletin.pdf (accessed 20 December 2021).
19. O'Hara R, Coster J, Goodacre S. Qualitative exploration of the Medical Examiner role in identifying problems with the quality of patient care. *BMJ Open.* 2021; 11: e048007.

CHAPTER 13

The Medical Examiner Service and Child Death Reviews

Nigel L Kennea

Introduction

Medical Examiners (MEs) should scrutinise all child deaths (under the age of 18 years) and contribute to accurate and timely completion of the Medical Certificate of Cause of Death (MCCD) or contribute to a coroner notification if necessary. Paediatric deaths have different patterns and aetiologies to those conditions affecting adults and so the ME may need to seek advice from paediatric colleagues to help with the scrutiny. Some Medical Examiner Services have found it helpful to employ an ME who is a senior paediatrician or neonatologist. Child deaths clearly involve a vulnerable population and are reviewed and reported though a number of systems. MEs and Medical Examiner Officers (MEOs) need to understand these systems and agree locally how to best interact with these other processes and help ensure families are supported in a consistent and sensitive way. Families will usually be directly supported by the clinical team involved, or through support provided by the child death overview panel (CDOP), with MEs having a 'light-touch' and not usually being the primary contact with the family. If at all possible, families should have a single point of contact to manage questions or concerns about clinical care. This would usually be a clinical team member soon after death, and then an allocated key worker from the CDOP following their review. Further information for MEs work in scrutinising child deaths is available in the recent National Medical Examiner's Good Practice Series No. 6.[1]

Patterns of Child Deaths

Child mortality can be subdivided into neonatal mortality (deaths below 28 days of age), infant mortality (deaths below 1 year of age) and child mortality, which includes deaths of all individuals up to their 18th birthday. There are approximately 5000 deaths in children aged 0–18 years each year in the UK, with 3347 child deaths occurring in England in the year to 31 March 2020.[2] There has been a decline in infant and child deaths in the last decades but the UK rates remain above those of many Western European countries. In 2012 more than 3000 children died before the age of 1. In 2019, there were 2390 infant deaths (under 1 year) and 907 deaths in children aged 1–15 years in England and Wales.[3] Both the

National Child Mortality Database (NCMD) and the Office for National Statistics (ONS) provide regular insights into the patterns of child death, and the NCMD now generates data and reports to inform understanding and learning. It is helpful for MEs to know the main learning from such reviews to help inform their thoughts on individual cases.

The second NCMD Annual Report[2] demonstrated that 42% of child deaths in England occurred below the age of 28 days with a high proportion occurring as a result of prematurity-related conditions, and 63% of child deaths occurred in the first year (Figure 13.1). More than half (56%) of all child deaths occurred in the two categories 'perinatal/neonatal' and 'chromosomal, genetic and congenital anomalies', with a large proportion occurring in the first year of life. All sudden unexpected, unexplained deaths require referral to the Coroner, as do those resulting from trauma or injury. The most frequent cause of death over 1 year of age relates to injury (Figure 13.2). The NCMD programme is attempting to identify 'modifiable factors' in a number of deaths and MEs should be aware of such data in scrutinising child deaths (Figure 13.3). Although the most frequent modifiable factor identified was smoking by a parent or carer, gaps in service delivery with challenges of access to services and poor communication were regularly identified. MEs need to be aware of any further investigations and reports related to child death. For example, the independent review of maternity services at Shrewsbury and Telford Hospital NHS Trust identified themes of poor care and missed opportunities for learning and improvement. MEs need to be aware of such reports in order to best support families and ensure focus on escalating concerns.[4] The importance of deprivation was highlighted with many more deaths in children from the most deprived neighbourhoods.

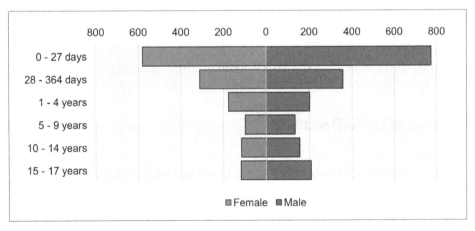

Figure 13.1   The number of child death notifications received by child death overview panels by age group and sex, year ending 31 March 2020.

Reproduced from: National Child Mortality Database Programme, Second Annual Report. Unadapted: Copyright © 2021 *Healthcare Quality Improvement Partnership. Reproduced with permission.*

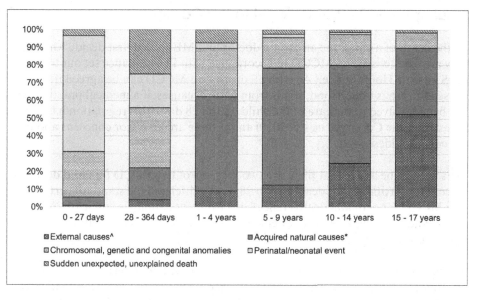

Figure 13.2 The proportion of reviews completed by child death overview panels in each age group by category of death, year ending 31 March 2020.

Reproduced from: National Child Mortality Database Programme, Second Annual Report. Unadapted: Copyright © 2021 Healthcare Quality Improvement Partnership. Reproduced with permission.

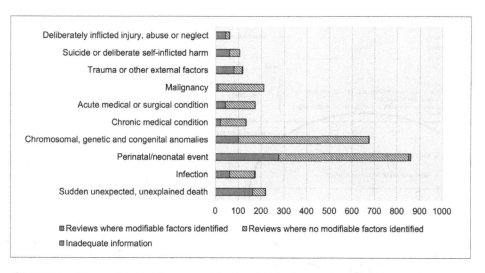

Figure 13.3 The number of reviews completed by child death overview panels by primary category of death and whether modifiable factors were identified, year ending 31 March 2020.

Reproduced from: National Child Mortality Database Programme, Second Annual Report. Unadapted: Copyright © 2021 Healthcare Quality Improvement Partnership. Reproduced with permission.

Issuing the MCCD or Referral to the Coroner

At the death of a child, the attending doctor and ME should first decide whether they are able to issue an MCCD in accordance with F66 guidance set out by the ONS and the Home Office.[5] As with all deaths, an MCCD can be agreed if the cause of death is understood, if it is from natural causes, if a medical practitioner has been involved in the care of the child within 28 days (this regulation has been adjusted in the Coronavirus Act 2020) and if there are no major concerns about the care provided.

MEs need to be aware that there are two versions of the MCCD for child deaths: a neonatal certificate (for deaths up to 28 days of life) and the standard certificate. The MCCD for neonatal deaths reflects the different aetiologies of death in this period and includes sections to document 'maternal diseases or conditions affecting infant' (Figures 13.4 and 6.1c and d).

It should be recognised that the deaths of children with long-term illnesses or life-limiting conditions, even when their death is anticipated, need to be individually scrutinised and it may still be necessary to refer the case to the Coroner if there are concerns, or the death meets other statutory criteria.

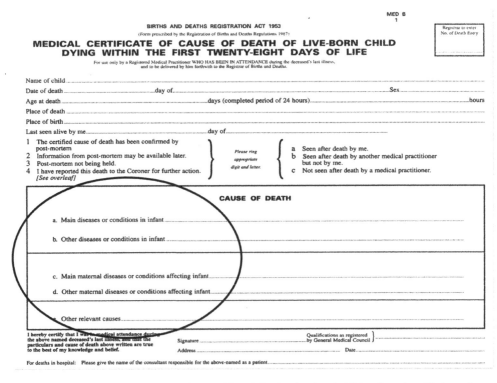

Figure 13.4 Medical certificate of Cause of Death for the deaths of children less than 28 days of age highlighting maternal/perinatal factors.

Attention should be given to how best to support the family through the process of registration and who is the best person to describe the wording on the MCCD to the family. In most cases this is best done by the clinical team caring for the child.

Interaction of Medical Examiner Services with other Child Death Reviews

There are already several processes for review of child deaths, and MEs need to understand them and establish relationships/contact with key individuals leading other processes, to ensure that questions, or learning, can be shared. In most cases, paediatric services will remain in contact with families in order to support them directly, with Medical Examiner Services contributing to helping the clinical teams in writing an accurate and timely MCCD, or aiding decisions related to Coroner referral. It is important that families have a single point of contact to raise questions or concerns rather than have individuals feeding back different information from separate review processes; this could be confusing, inconsistent and upsetting. It should be acknowledged that different review processes occur with different professional groups, over different timescales, and so managing this can be exceptionally challenging. It is important that the family 'voice' is heard in all investigations and that learning is shared.

Child Death Overview Panels and National Child Mortality Database (NCMD)

The Children Act (2004) required local authorities in England to review the death of every child in England to determine whether there were any modifiable factors that could lead to system improvements. Local child death overview panels (CDOPs) were created with the purpose of investigating the circumstances of death of every child in their region. Although helpful, it was acknowledged that there was considerable variability in how CDOPs worked and functioned in their first years, and so, following the Children and Social Work Act (2017) and subsequent Statutory and Operational Guidance 2018,[6] reforms were made to provide greater consistency to the child death review process and help the experience of bereaved families. Local authorities and commissioning groups are now required to come together to form child death review partnerships and take joint ownership and oversight of child deaths within their region.

This CDOP process in England demands that an independent review of the case must be carried out for all children under 18 years of age regardless of the cause of death. This includes any live-born baby. The CDOPs do not review cases of stillborn infants where there was a healthcare professional in attendance. CDOPs are set up to cover a geographic area and review the deaths of children resident in that area. CDOP notifications should occur within 24 hours of death. The panel's review is multi-professional with contributions from professionals directly involved in the care of the deceased, and professionals involved in the investigation into the death. It is helpful for MEs and MEOs to understand their local CDOP structure and be aware of the leaders/points of contact. Although it is the clinical team's responsibility to notify the CDOP of a child death, the ME may identify issues that should be included in the CDOP notification and discuss them with the clinical team involved. Also, Medical Examiner Services might help remind clinical teams about the CDOP referral process in the rare event that children (less than 18 years) die in an adult care setting less familiar with child death processes. Paediatricians should be aware of the local processes, and the timely reporting of deaths to CDOP using standard forms. The notifications provide further information about the child in the context of their family and collects health and social information, including details of safeguarding issues. As with the scrutiny of all vulnerable patients, MEs need to consider safeguarding concerns when liaising and discussing cases with the attending clinicians. For each CDOP case review, a key worker should be allocated as a point of contact who can provide information and updates and signpost sources of support.

The nature of CDOP meetings and investigation will vary according to the circumstances. CDOP notifications should occur as soon after death as possible, and within 24 hours. A rapid joint agency response (including involvement of health professionals, a police investigator and social services) should be triggered if the death: *'is or could be due to external causes; is sudden and there is no immediately apparent cause; occurs in custody, or where the child was detained under the Mental Health Act; where the initial circumstances raise any suspicions that the death may not have been natural; or in the case of a stillbirth where no healthcare professional was in attendance'.*[6]

The ME needs to be aware of the review and develop relationships with clinical teams and local CDOP panels (all have a designated doctor) and ensure that there is accurate completion of MCCD, or appropriate referral to the Coroner, and that all understand who is the main point of contact for a given family to ensure good support and accurate communication. It is useful if the main point of contact can provide information about the MES and can inform the family that they may be contacted.

Information from CDOPs is sent to the National Child Mortality Database (NCMD), which analyses/interprets trends in order to derive and share learning. Although MEs are unlikely to interact with the NCMD directly, MEs should be aware of their publications, current trends and potential learning identified, as it may be relevant to case scrutiny and may inform learning from individual deaths.

Perinatal Mortality Review Tool (PMRT)

In addition to CDOP processes, there is a further local review process for neonatal deaths. The Perinatal Mortality Review Tool (PMRT) process is multi-professional and includes input from different care settings related to perinatal management. The PMRT uses a web-based tool that is designed to support a standardised review of care of perinatal deaths in neonatal units from 22+0 weeks' gestation to 28 days after birth. It is also available to support the review of post-neonatal deaths where the baby dies in a neonatal unit after 28 days but has never left hospital following birth. At clinicians' discretion it might also be used for the review of deaths of live-born infants of less than 22+0 weeks' gestation, where a death certificate has been issued. The PMRT is integrated with the national collection of perinatal mortality surveillance data. MEs would not usually be involved in the PMRT process but they may point out potential issues for PMRT consideration in their discussion with the clinical team. In some circumstances the ME might be interested in the outcome of the PMRT for a specific case and therefore relationships with key clinical staff leading obstetric and neonatal governance are very helpful.

Healthcare Safety Investigation Branch (HSIB)

The Healthcare Safety Investigation Branch (HSIB) conducts independent investigations of patient safety concerns in NHS-funded care across England. It independently investigates incidents that meet the 'Each Baby Counts' criteria. 'Each Baby Counts' is the Royal College of Obstetricians and Gynaecologists' national quality improvement programme designed to reduce the number of babies who die or are left severely disabled as a result of incidents occurring during term labour.[5] It investigates early neonatal deaths related to labour and delivery and any death within the first week of life (0–6 days) of any cause. The HSIB investigations require family consent and have direct family support. The HSIB conducts interviews and gathers information from multi-professional teams. It looks into all clinical and medical aspects of the incident, as well as aspects of the workplace environment and culture surrounding the incident. It is not likely that MEs will be engaged in HSIB investigations, but it is important they know of the process and important outcomes.

Learning Disability Mortality Review Programme and Child Death

The NHS Long Term Plan[8] made a commitment to review deaths in people with learning disabilities and autism, and to use the information to improve health and wellbeing. As well as reviewing adult patients, all deaths of children over the age of 4 years with learning disability or autism should be referred to the LeDeR programme for review. Any professional can notify the LeDeR programme of a death.[9] MEs need to be aware of their local processes and contacts for Learning from Deaths (LfD) and LeDeR coordinators and may help in identifying cases to report.

Conclusions

The patterns of death in children are different to adult deaths and so MEs may require input from specialists. Differing patterns of child death are reflected in a separate MCCD for neonatal deaths (less than 28 days). Generally, ME services will not be the 'point of contact' for bereaved families in child death, but they should be aware of several other mortality review processes in order to feed information into them, or to gain insights from them to aid future scrutiny. ME services are well placed to identify cases to local Learning from Deaths coordinators or those involved in notification to LeDeR. ME services need to scrutinise child deaths in a similar way to other patients and work very closely with clinical teams to ensure timely, accurate and consistent MCCDs, or referral to the Coroner.

REFERENCES

1. National Medical Examiner's Good Practice Series No. 1 www.rcpath.org/uploads/assets/7fa7a9d6-ada5-4597-b16f4602c93d3e91/Good-Practice-Series-Child-Deaths.pdf (accessed 22 June 22).
2. National Child Mortality Database. NCMD Second Annual Report, 2021. https://www.ncmd.info/publications/2nd-annual-report/ (accessed 20 December 2021).
3. Office for National Statistics. Child and Infant Mortality in England and Wales: 2019, 2021. https://www.ons.gov.uk/peoplepopulationandcommunity/birthsdeathsandmarriages/deaths/bulletins/childhoodinfantandperinatalmortalityinenglandandwales/2019 (accessed 20 December 2021).
4. Office for National Statistics. Guidance for Doctors Completing Medical Certificates of Cause of Death in England and Wales, 2020. https://assets.publishing.service.gov.uk/government/uploads/system/uploads/attachment_data/file/877302/guidance-for-doctors-completing-medical-certificates-of-cause-of-death-covid-19.pdf (accessed 20 December 2021).
5. Ockenden D. Findings, conclusions and essential actions from the independent review of maternity services at The Shrewsbury and Telford Hospital NHS Trust published 30 March 2022. www.ockendenmaternityreview.org.uk (accessed 22 June 2022).
6. GOV.uk. Child Death Review. Statutory and Operational Guidance (England), 2018. https://assets.publishing.service.gov.uk/government/uploads/system/uploads/attachment_data/file/859302/child-death-review-statutory-and-operational-guidance-england.pdf (accessed 20 December 2021).
7. Royal College of Obstetricians and Gynaecologists. Each Baby Counts: 2020 Final Progress Report, 2020. https://www.rcog.org.uk/en/guidelines-research-services/audit-quality-improvement/each-baby-counts/reports-updates/2020-report/ (accessed 20 December 2021).
8. NHS England. NHS Long Term Plan, 2020. https://www.longtermplan.nhs.uk/ (accessed 20 December 2021).
9. NHS England. Report the Death of Someone with a Learning Disability. https://leder.nhs.uk/report (accessed 20 December 2021).

CHAPTER 14

Law and Procedures Related to Burial and Cremation

Nigel Callaghan and Gabriel Callaghan

Introduction

In this chapter, we discuss relevant laws surrounding burial and cremation. We start with the contentious question of 'who owns a body after death'. Then, we provide a brief background surrounding burial legislation. The laws and procedures relating to cremation are considerably more detailed than those for burial. We discuss how a crematorium operates and the process of applying for a cremation. We discuss the cremation forms and provide advice on how to complete them correctly. Finally, we discuss the role of the Home Office medical referee.

Who Owns a Body after Death?

'There is no property in a dead body, but a common law duty to arrange for its proper disposal.' This duty falls primarily on the personal representatives of the deceased person.[1] What does this mean? A dead body is owned by no one. However, an executor of probate (the legal right to deal with an estate) acts as the agent of the deceased person, with the rights and obligations starting on death. Following cremation, the next of kin do not own the ashes, but have possession of them. When there is a dispute, the courts will usually rule in favour of the wishes of the deceased as regards to how their body is disposed of, following the case of Burrows v HM Coroner for Preston, in which Jason Smith stated that *'in as much as our domestic law says that the views of a deceased person can be ignored is no longer good law'*.[2] Table 14.1 shows the priority of beneficial interest in the death estate under the Non-Contentious Probate Rules 1987.

Possession in law is not the same as ownership. A hospital has a right to detain a body if it is infectious. Then, the Coroner can take temporary possession of a body to determine the cause of death, and thereafter, following the examination, the body is released to the appropriate person, who is usually the executor of the will. Legally, there is no obligation to use a funeral director and funeral directors are largely unregulated (see Chapter 16). If no one claims responsibility for the

DOI: 10.1201/9781003188759-14

Table 14.1 Priority of beneficial interest in the death estate under the Non-Contentious Probate Rules 1987

1. The surviving husband and wife
2. The children of the deceased
3. The mother and father of the deceased
4. Brothers and sisters of the whole blood and the issue of any deceased brother or sister of the whole blood who died before the deceased
5. Brothers and sisters of the half blood and the issue of any deceased brother or sister of the half-blood who died before the deceased
6. Grandparents
7. Uncles and aunts of the whole blood and the issue of any deceased uncle or aunt of the whole blood who died before the deceased
8. Uncles and aunts of the half blood and the issue of any deceased uncle or aunt of the half-blood who died before the deceased

body, and there are limited means to pay, then the local authority is responsible for burial or cremation. In extraordinary circumstances related to a health risk to others, a magistrate can order steps to be taken to secure the burial or cremation of the body under the Public Health (Control of Disease) Act 1984.

The view that a body is not property in law does not preclude theft charges if a body is stolen and something is done with it. One case, in 1998, involved an artist who stole body parts from the Royal College of Surgeons to make macabre sculptures and exhibit them.[3] The judge ruled that the common law principle still stands, but that *'parts of a corpse are capable of being property within section 4 of the Theft Act 1968 if they have acquired different attributes by virtue of the application of skill'*. This means that a prosecution under the Theft Act 1968 can be brought if 'body parts' acquire different attributes by the application of skill.

On occasion, the disposal of a body can be contentious, and the courts become involved. Medical Examiners may encounter contentions between family members. One recent dispute between three daughters and a niece involved the determination of whether the body should be buried in the UK or Jamaica, and what the wishes of the deceased were.[4] An injunction was granted to prohibit the disposal of the body until a hearing could be arranged to determine the appropriate party to dispose of the body.

Burial Laws

Before 1852, there were limited laws surrounding burial. However, the Burial Act 1852 (with various amendments) was introduced as the population increased. The burial laws were separated into temporal (non-Church of England) and ecclesiastical (Church of England) laws. In the modern day, ecclesiastical ground is consecrated with special rules. Ecclesiastical offences (church offences) can be committed during a burial on consecrated land – for example, a church graveyard – such as wrongful exhumation and 'riotous or indecent behaviour'.

Local authorities operate many cemeteries and have responsibilities in law. These are defined in the Local Authorities Cemeteries Order 1977, which details their responsibilities for keeping accurate records surrounding the occupants of a grave. Local authorities have the power to do *all such things as they consider necessary or desirable for the proper management*. Generally, a local authority will lease a grave to an applicant for a period of 25–100 years. If the lease is not renewed, graves can be re-used after 75 years.

There is no law explicitly prohibiting a body from being buried on private land, provided that the death is appropriately registered, and there is an appropriate burial register to reference where the body is buried. Environmental laws need to be considered during a private burial. However, it is an offence to outrage public modesty when burying a body.

Lawful and decent burial of a body

Any person who acts to prevent the 'lawful and decent burial of a body' is guilty of an indictable criminal offence under common law. In 2012, a multi-millionaire was handed a custodial sentence for keeping the body of his deceased wife in his house without a proper burial for over two months.[5] The body was decomposing in the house and had been kept under bin bags sealed with gaffer tape. In 1986, a criminal offence was committed when a drug addict died in a flat and their cohabitants rolled the deceased's body in carpet and disposed of it in a quarry. It is a criminal offence to detain a body for payment (e.g. the funeral director cannot detain a body due to fees not being paid), as this would prevent the decent burial of the body. Burials must not outrage public modesty under common law; in other words, bodies must be buried in a dignified manner. An example of an undignified manner would be putting a naked body on display.

Exhumation of a body

Exhumation is the re-opening of a grave to remove an object, remove the body or examine the body. This can occur if further enquiries after death are required, or the body is to be cremated. An application for exhumation must be made under section 25 of the Burial Act 1857. On consecrated ground controlled by the Church of England, an application to the consistory court of the diocese is required.

Background to Cremation

In the UK, 78.45% of people who died in 2020 were cremated.[6] Cremation regulations are in addition to the registration of death regulations. The Cremation (England and Wales) Regulations 2008 define the law surrounding cremation. This section describes how a crematorium operates, outlines cremation regulations, advises how to complete the forms and explains the role of the crematorium medical referee. Medical Examiners (MEs) and Medical Examiners Officers (MEOs) should be aware of the principles surrounding cremation as this may assist in discussions with the bereaved.

How does a crematorium operate?

Crematoriums (or crematoria) are often operated by local authorities, although an increasing number are privately owned. There is no law requiring someone to use a funeral director; however, the crematorium used must be appropriately licenced. The next of kin can make an application directly to the crematorium and obtain the relevant medical certificates for the body to be cremated. However, the funeral director will usually be responsible for arranging the completion of the forms.

Immediately after a death, the body will be stored in a hospital mortuary if the death occurred in hospital. If the body is not detained by the Coroner, it can be received by the funeral director (if the next of kin has one) or the next of kin. The process of preparing the body for cremation can then take place.

To prevent harmful emissions, there are regulations surrounding what a body can be dressed in when it is prepared for cremation, although sophisticated filtering systems are present in modern crematoriums. The body can be dressed or remain naked, but it must not be fitted with any harmful or dangerous devices (such as battery-powered watches). Certain items can be left in a coffin, such as wooden rosary beads and written messages; however, there should be nothing combustible in the coffin, such as alcohol. Some materials are not suitable for cremation, such as plastic or fibreglass coffins, although others, such as wicker, are. Crematoria can advise on industry standard guidelines.

Funeral services are often conducted in crematoriums, although the service can be held elsewhere, and the body subsequently transported to the crematorium. At the end of the service in a crematorium, the curtains are closed and the door behind the curtains in the chapel or multi-faith room leads to the cremator area. Usually, bodies are cremated on the same day as the service. The time to cremate a body depends on the size of the body, but it generally takes between one and three hours.

When the crematorium attendant receives a coffin, they first check the nameplate on the coffin, and cross-reference this with the electronic database and cremation documentation to check that the cremation has been correctly authorised. They then load the coffin into the cremator, entering the identity of the deceased into the computer and attaching the form to the same cremator in which the body is being cremated, to ensure that the relatives receive the correct ashes. The body is then

cremated. The crematorium attendant will then rake all the ashes and any uncre-
mated bones into an urn, which mitigates the risk of ashes being spilled on the
floor. Care and attention is paid to this task, to ensure that all of the remains of the
deceased person are extracted. The ID of the deceased person always remains with
the ashes, to ensure relatives receive the correct ashes. Occasionally, there may be
some bone fragments left. These are inserted into the cremulator (a machine that
reduces larger fragments to fine ash) to be ground down. Finally, all of the ashes
are ready for the family to bury or scatter.

Who can apply for a cremation?

Under Regulation 15 of the Cremation (England and Wales) Regulations 2008,
an executor of the estate or a near relative can apply for a cremation. In the
regulations, a 'near relative' means a widow, widower, surviving partner, parent, child or any other relative usually residing with the deceased person. The
crematorium medical referee (CMR) can also authorise a cremation if a fit and
proper person makes the application and there is a good reason why the application is not made by an executor or near relative.

Who can receive the ashes?

Disputes often arise around who has the right to collect the ashes. There was
previously some ambiguity around this in the law, but this was cleared up by the
Cremation (England and Wales) (Amendment) Regulations 2017. Legally, a crematorium must dispose of the ashes in accordance with the instructions from the
applicant. If the applicant does not want the ashes, the crematorium must retain
the ashes and 'decently inter the ashes in the ground or scatter them'. Before the crematorium does this, it must give 14 days' notice to the applicant.

If disposal becomes contentious, the courts can become involved, and will issue an
injunction (e.g. an order for the crematorium to give the ashes to someone).

A crematorium cannot retain ashes for payment.

Medical Cremation Forms

Incorrectly completed cremation forms can cause a cremation to be delayed and
can cause substantial distress to a family. This section explains how the forms
should be completed. These forms are in addition to any Medical Certificate
of Cause of Death (MCCD), which is required for registration of the death, as
discussed in Chapter 6. All cremation forms must be completed legibly, all relevant questions must be answered, and questions should be completed in full.
Abbreviations should be avoided.

Cremation forms are in a standardised format, given in amendments to the 2008 Cremation Regulations. If the standard forms are not used, the cremation may not be authorised. Whenever a question is not applicable, 'not applicable' should be written. Guidance is available for completing Cremation Form 4.[7]

The applicant to the cremation has the right under the regulations to inspect the forms. However, there may be 'harmful information' that is relevant to the form, such as a sexually transmitted infection, and this is something the doctor should consider when completing the form. If there is any potentially 'harmful information', then consideration should be given to not writing this information on the form itself but adding an extra sheet marked 'in confidence' for the attention of the medical referee.

It is important to note that these forms are legal documents, and it is a criminal offence to make a dishonest declaration. In 2018, a doctor was struck off the medical register and criminally convicted for signing 485 forms without proper scrutiny.[8]

Cremation Form 4

Cremation Form 4 (medical certificate) must be completed by a 'registered medical practitioner', which means a medical doctor registered with the General Medical Council with a licence to practice (not a nurse or other healthcare professional). This could be the same doctor who completes the MCCD, referred to as the 'certificate required for the registration of death' on Cremation Form 4. They must complete this form themselves and cannot delegate its completion to someone else. There is no requirement of tenure for the doctor signing Cremation Form 4.

Question 5 on the form is 'Were you the deceased's usual medical practitioner?'. The usual medical practitioner is normally the deceased's GP, although if the deceased was an in-patient in hospital for a length of time, then this could be taken to be the 'hospital medical practitioner' who attended the deceased.

A doctor should only complete Cremation Form 4 if they attended the deceased during their last illness within 14 days before death. If these conditions are not met, then the form should be completed by a doctor who did attend the deceased, or the death should be referred to the Coroner. These conditions are tested by questions 6 and 7 on the form. These conditions can only be deviated from in exceptional circumstances.

The cause of death in question 11 should be the same as that on the MCCD. The medical referee must be satisfied that the cause of death has been definitely ascertained. To enable this, the medical referee will evaluate the cause of death from the cremation forms and determine whether the cause of death fits with the other information provided on the form and if the cause is logical. When the medical referee requires further information, they will contact the doctor signing the form and they may obtain medical records. If the cause of death is deemed 'unascertained', the Coroner must be informed of the death.

On any question requiring the name and contact information of any person (persons who were present at death and contact details of medical staff), details must be provided in a format that will enable the doctor completing Cremation Form 5 and the medical referee to contact them if further questions remain surrounding the cause of death. Failure to do this can cause unnecessary delays.

The Notification of Death Regulations 2019[9] set out when a death must be reported to the Coroner. This includes the following circumstances:

1. If there is a suspicion that the death was unnatural
2. If there is a suspicion that the death was violent
3. If the cause of death is not known
4. If the deceased had a disease that must be notified to the Coroner
5. If no medical practitioner attended the deceased within the last 14 days of their life
6. If the death occurred while the deceased was in state detention
7. If the cause of death was related to the deceased's occupation.

The outcome of the communication with the Coroner must be recorded in questions 20 and 21 of Cremation Form 4. Ministry of Justice statistics show that 40% of all deaths in England and Wales were reported to a Coroner in 2019. Of these, 39% of deaths referred underwent a post-mortem examination and 14% of referred cases resulted in an inquest.[10]

Before the 'statement of truth', a final question regards 'hazardous implants' that could pose a risk of danger to the crematorium staff or the crematorium. If a pacemaker was left in the body, it could cause an explosion. In 2011, there was an explosion in a crematorium in Grenoble that had enough force to fire a 16lb artillery shell at 60mph, and extensive damage was caused. Research was conducted to further investigate pacemaker explosions.[11] Table 14.2 lists examples of hazardous implants and materials that need to be declared and removed.

Removal can be done by mortuary staff. There is no requirement that the removal is done by a doctor.

Cremation Form 5

Cremation Form 5 is now only of historic interest. This cremation certificate has now been permanently removed. It was temporarily removed as an easement by

Table 14.2 Implants listed by the Cremation (England and Wales) Regulations 2008 (Annex A) that could cause problems during cremation

- Pacemakers
- Implantable cardioverter defibrillators (ICDs)
- Cardiac resynchronisation therapy devices (CRTDs)
- Implantable loop recorders
- Ventricular assist devices (VADs): left ventricular assist devices (LVADs); right ventricular assist devices (RVADs); or biventricular assist devices BiVADs)
- Implantable drug pumps including intrathecal pumps
- Neurostimulators (including for pain and functional electrical stimulation)
- Bone growth stimulators
- Hydrocephalus programmable shunts
- Fixion nails
- Any other battery powered or pressurised implant
- Radioactive implants
- Radiopharmaceutical treatment (via injection)

the Coronavirus Act 2020 but since the expiry of the Act this change has been made permanent. The purpose of Cremation Form 5 (confirmatory medical certificate) was to add scrutiny to the facts given by the doctor who signed Cremation Form 4, that is: is the sequence of events leading to the death logical?

The Cremation Form 5 had stricter conditions on who can complete it than form 4. Form 5 had to be completed by a 'registered medical practitioner of at least 'five years standing', meaning that they must have held a full licence to practise for at least five years. Additionally, a doctor completing Form 5 could not be a relative of the deceased or of the doctor signing Form 4, and must not be a relative, partner or close colleague of anyone in the same clinical team as the doctor signing Form 4. If a Cremation Form 5 was not completed by a doctor meeting the necessary criteria, then the medical referee would reject the form, and this could delay the funeral.

A Cremation Form 5 was not required where the death occurred in a hospital where the deceased was an in-patient and there was a post-mortem examination of the body, and where the post-mortem was performed or supervised by a doctor with at least five years standing.

The doctor completing Form 5 had to question the doctor who completed Form 4 to ascertain the reasonableness of the conclusions made by the doctor who completed Form 4.

Other questions in Part 2 of Cremation Form 5 discussed potential lines of inquiry for the doctor completing it. The doctor had to speak to at least one other person with knowledge of the deceased, either another doctor who attended them, someone who nursed the deceased during their last illness or was present at the time of death, a member of the deceased's family or another person (relationship to be explained on the form). If at least one of these interactions was not recorded the medical referee would reject the form.

Cremation Forms under the Coronavirus Act 2020

The regulations surrounding completion of the forms during the SARS-CoV-2 pandemic were changed for the duration of the emergency legislation which expired on 24th March 2022. The key changes to the regulations were:

1. Cremation Form 5 was not required.
2. The acceptable period before death for not being seen by a medical practitioner for Form 4 was increased from 14 days to 28 days. This condition was replaced with '*either seen the patient 28 days before death or has examined the body after death*'.
3. Any medical practitioner could sign Cremation Form 4, even if they have not attended the deceased during their last illness or after death, provided that the below conditions were satisfied:
   i) The medical practitioner who did attend the deceased is unable to sign Cremation Form 4 or it is impractical for them to do so; and
   ii) A medical practitioner has seen the deceased (including audio-visual/video consultation) within 28 days before death or has viewed the body in person after death.

The circumstances in which another doctor could complete the MCCD, and Cremation Form 4 is a moot point, but legally this implied some significant barrier preventing the doctor signing the form, such as the doctor being incapacitated through illness, or self-isolating due to a positive COVID-19 test or close contact with someone with the infection. This part of the rule was interpreted differently in different ME Services, with some MEs completing MCCDs when the attending doctor is unavailable due to caring for patients or being on leave for any reason. In some hospitals the MEs completed all MCCDs and Cremation Form 4s.

Following expiry of the Act on 24 March 2022 the following provisions relevant to cremation were retained:

- the period before death within which a doctor completing an MCCD (medical certificate of cause of death) should see a deceased patient will remain 28 days
- it will still be acceptable for medical practitioners to send MCCDs to registrars electronically
- the form Cremation 5 will not be re-introduced
- the temporary provision allowing any medical practitioner to complete the MCCD will be discontinued.

The Role of the Crematorium Medical Referee

Crematorium medical referees are appointed for each cremation authority by the secretary of state. Some medical referees are contracted by the local authority, which pays them, since many crematoriums are operated by the public sector.

Under the Cremation Regulations, a medical referee must be a 'registered medical practitioner' with at least 'five years of standing'. In the regulations, these conditions are defined as a doctor who has been fully registered for five years, although they typically have far more than five years' experience.

What is the role of a crematorium medical referee?

No cremation can take place unless the medical referee authorises it via a Cremation Form 10. The questions that the medical referee must be satisfied about are:

1. The requirements of the Cremation (England and Wales) Regulations 2008 are satisfied.
2. The inquiry made by the persons who gave the relevant certificates (Form 4 and Form 5) are accurate.
3. The fact and cause of death have been definitely ascertained, or if not, a Coroner has been informed and has given permission for the body to be disposed of (e.g. by opening an inquest or issuing a Form 100A).

To 'definitely ascertain' the cause of death is a far higher standard than for a burial. This is because exhumation of ashes is less feasible than a buried body, and limited information can be obtained from ashes.

If a death is referred to the Coroner, information about the outcome of the Coroner's investigation must be given. For example, the Coroner may issue a Form 100A and instruct the certifying doctor to issue the MCCD, in which case there is no post-mortem examination or inquest. If the Coroner decides to investigate further, Cremation Forms 4 and 5 are not required, and a Cremation Form 6 is provided by the Coroner to indicate that they have no need for any further examination of the body.

How Does a Medical Referee Work?

The medical referee is contracted by the local crematorium, so there is no need for the applicant to find a suitably qualified medical referee. Often, the medical referee will attend the crematorium in person to inspect the forms delivered by the funeral director, although, increasingly, electronically completed forms are reviewed remotely. The medical referee will critically evaluate the forms to ensure that adequate enquiries have been made about the cause of death. The medical referee has the legal authority to make their own enquiries, although they are not compelled to do so if they are satisfied.

These enquiries may include contacting the doctor who completed Cremation Forms 4 and 5 to ascertain the rationale behind the assertions made. The medical referee may contact those present at the death to corroborate any information. This is why it is crucial to provide appropriate contact details when completing the forms.

The medical referee has a power under Regulation 24 of the Cremation Regulations (England and Wales) 2008 to order a post-mortem examination of the body by an appropriately qualified person who is licensed under section 16 of the Human Tissue Act 2004, if they deem it necessary. This occurs very rarely, as, if there is any doubt that the cause of death was natural or the cause of death is not known, the case would be referred to the Coroner. It is rare for a cremation not to be authorised, and the medical referee must provide the applicant with written reasons.

Why Do Medical Referees Reject Forms?

It is not the role of the medical referee to exert power over the doctor completing the cremation forms, but to critically assess the assertions that are made. Wherever possible, the medical referee will work with the doctor to minimise distress to the family of the deceased. Common reasons for rejecting forms are:

1. Ineligibility of the signing doctor, either because they didn't attend the deceased during their last illness, haven't seen them within 28 days or after death, or the only recent consultation was by phone.
2. Illegible handwriting. If handwriting is an issue, forms can be typed or completed electronically.
3. Inappropriate completion of questions, e.g. stating 'natural causes' rather than providing sufficient detail about the actual conditions that led to the death.
4. Non-completion of questions, e.g. not stating when you last saw the deceased or omitting sections of the form rather than stating 'not applicable'.
5. Not answering the question about hazardous implants.
6. Not referring cases to the Coroner when the cause of death is notifiable.

The Future of the Cremation System and Crematorium Medical Referee

The initial intention was that cremation forms and the role of the CMR would be abolished when the statutory Medical Examiner system was introduced. CMRs were first informed of this by the Ministry of Justice in 2012, and all referees appointed since then have been made aware of the intention to eventually abolish the role. The government's consultation into the impact of ME implementation[11] identified concerns about how some aspects of the CMR role would be covered and stated that the issue would be revisited in due course. The timescales for removing Cremation Form 4 and ceasing the role of CMRs is not yet known. Currently, the future of the Medical Referee is uncertain. The Cremation Regulations are different from the Health and Social Care Act 2022 so abolishing the role would require changes to the legislation by parliament. However, as a Medical Examiner, the elements of good practice developed over more than a decade of the Medical Referee role should be transferrable to the Medical Examiner role.

REFERENCES

1. Buchanan v Milton. 2 FLR 844, 1999.
2. Burrows v HM Coroner for Preston. EWHC 1387 (QB), 2008.
3. R v Kelly and Lindsay. 3 All E.R. 741, 1998.
4. Anstey v Mundle & Anor. EWHC 1073 (Ch), 2016.
5. BBC News. Rausing Sentenced for Delaying Wife Eva's Burial, 2012. https://www.bbc.co.uk/news/uk-england-london-19078646 (accessed 20 December 2021).
6. The Cremation Society. Progress of Cremation in the British Islands from 1885 to 2020. https://www.cremation.org.uk/progress-of-cremation-united-kingdom (accessed 20 December 2021).
7. Ministry of Justice. The Cremation (England and Wales) Regulations 2008. Guidance to medical practitioners completing form Cremation 4. March 2022 https://assets.publishing.service.gov.uk/government/uploads/system/uploads/attachment_data/file/1062509/medical-practitioners-completing-form-cremation-4-25-march-2022.pdf
8. Dyer C. Consultant who signed cremation forms without examining the bodies is struck off. *BMJ*. 2020; 371: 4846.
9. GOV.uk. The Notification of Death Regulations, 2019. https://www.legislation.gov.uk/uksi/2019/1112/contents/made (accessed 20 December 2021).
10. Ministry of Justice. Coroner Statistics Annual 2019, England and Wales, 2020. https://assets.publishing.service.gov.uk/government/uploads/system/uploads/attachment_data/file/888314/Coroners_Statistics_Annual_2019_.pdf (accessed 20 December 2021).
11. Gale C, Mulley G. Pacemaker explosions in crematoria: problems and possible solutions. *JRSM*. 2002; 95(7): 353–355.
12. Department of Health AND Social Care. Introduction of Medical Examiners and Reforms to Death Certification in England and Wales: Government Response to Consultation, 2018. https://assets.publishing.service.gov.uk/government/uploads/system/uploads/attachment_data/file/715224/death-certification-reforms-government-response.pdf (accessed 20 December 2021).

CHAPTER 15

Faith Implications of the Medical Examiner System

Mohamed Omer, Chandu Tailor and Daniel Elton

Introduction

The 2011 census (the 2021 census is scheduled to be published piecemeal between June 2022 and Summer 2023) reported that despite falling numbers, Christianity remained the largest religion in England and Wales with 33.2 million people (59.3% of the population). The second largest religious group were Muslims with 2.7 million people (4.8% of the population), having grown in the previous decade (2001–2010). The proportion of the population who reported they had no religion was ~25% of the population, while 7.2% of people did not answer the question in the census.[1] The proportion of other minority religious groups is shown in Figure 15.1.

In 2011, London was the most diverse region, with the highest proportions of people identifying as Muslim, Buddhist, Hindu and Jewish. The north-east and north-west of England had the highest proportion of Christians, and Wales had the highest proportion of people reporting no religion. In terms of local authorities, Knowsley had the highest proportion of people reporting to be Christians (80.9%) and Tower Hamlets had the highest proportion of Muslims (34.5%, more than seven times the average figure for England and Wales). Norwich had the highest proportion of the population reporting no religion (42.5%).

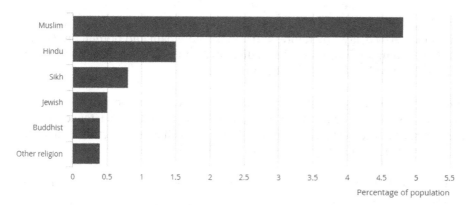

Figure 15.1 Minority religious groups in England and Wales in 2011.[1]

DOI: 10.1201/9781003188759-15

This chapter looks at the needs of the Muslim, Hindu, Sikh and Jewish communities, although many of the issues raised will apply to other faith and non-faith groups.

Muslims and the Medical Examiner System

'*Every soul shall taste death*' (3.185)

Muslims believe that they have been sent to this temporary world to prepare for a life of eternity, which begins when they die and leave this world. The Prophet Muhammad (peace be upon him) was sent to this world as a guide to how Muslims should live their lives from the day they are born to the time they depart from this world.

Due to the inevitability of death, Muslims of all ages are encouraged to talk about death and therefore it is not a taboo subject in the community. Muslims are constantly reminded about death and are encouraged to visit the cemetery frequently so that death can be remembered.

It is extremely important for Muslims that they bury their loved ones as soon as possible. A timeframe of 24 hours is commonly given; however, this is just a guide. The requirement is that the deceased are buried as soon as possible (in less than 24 hours if possible). Whilst this may not be possible in some cases due to the legal process that needs to be adhered to, Muslims request that all those who are involved in the process of death and end-of-life recognise that this is a fundamental belief. Any assistance that can be provided to ensure that the deceased are buried as soon as possible is greatly appreciated.

It is very common that whenever someone dies from the Muslim community, the family and friends will offer their condolences to the loved ones of the deceased. More often than not, the next question will be, 'when will the burial take place?' This is indicative of the importance attached to a speedy burial.

In reality, the family members cannot begin the grieving process until the burial takes place. Any delays, therefore, will impose more pain and burden on the family members and in some cases, tradition dictates that those who come to pay their respects must be looked after by the family members.

Why do Muslims hasten to bury their loved ones? According to religious texts, if a person has been an obedient servant of Allah, they should be hastened to their grave so that they can start to reap the reward of all their good actions, and if they have been disobedient, they will have to face the consequences.

Before a Muslim is buried, there are five processes they need to go through, and these are shown in Table 15.1.

Table 15.1   The five processes a Muslim needs to go through after death

1. Washing	The body must undergo a ritual wash (Ghusl), which is essential to ensure that any impurities are removed. The general ruling is that men should carry out the washing of other men and women should wash women, except a child under the age of 2 who can be washed by either sex. It is deemed a great reward to participate in this noble deed and as such, family members are encouraged to participate if they are able to do so.
2. Shrouding	Once the ritual wash is complete, the body is shrouded in three sheets of plain material for men and five sheets for women.
3. Final prayer	The final congregational prayer (Salaatul Janazah) for the deceased is compulsory, and it is a right of one Muslim over another.
4. Transportation of the deceased to their final resting place	If possible, it is recommended that the attendees carry the bier to the burial place.
5. Burial	Muslims are only permitted shroud burials. Only in exceptional circumstances are coffin burials permitted, such as when there is fear of a highly infectious disease being transmitted to others.

Not only must the necessary paperwork for burial be issued, but all the steps in Table 15.1 also need to take place before the burial process is complete. Thus, Muslims request that all those who are involved in the legal process fulfil their duties in a timely and efficient manner.

Muslims regard the human body (alive or dead) as sacrosanct and therefore do not permit the desecration of the body in any way. Hence, post-mortem examinations are not permitted, unless legally required. Where a post-mortem is deemed necessary, Coroners are requested to offer bereaved families an option for a non-invasive post-mortem where appropriate, and this has been recognised by the Chief Coroner in his guidance.[2]

The Muslim community welcomes the Medical Examiner (ME) system and appreciates the reason for its introduction.

The Muslim community recognises that the new ME system may bring benefits for the bereaved families, such as:

1. Fewer cases will be referred to the Coroner. This has been confirmed in pilot centres.
2. Improved quality of the Medical Certificate of Cause of Death (MCCD), reducing the likelihood of the MCCD being rejected by the registrar and causing further delays and distress to the family.
3. More accountability for the treatment and care provided to patients.
4. MEs being used to issue the MCCD in community deaths where the patient's general practitioner (GP) is not available, and other doctors from the practice are not able to issue a MCCD.

Medical Examiners also have a discussion with the family about the MCCD before it is issued, to ensure that families have an opportunity to ask any questions or raise any concerns. The bereaved families' main priority is the issuance of the MCCD so that the burial can proceed, and often this is done by a representative of the deceased's family. The community would urge flexibility in the system to allow the conversation with the ME to take place after the MCCD has been issued (perhaps up to a few days later).

Ideally, the Muslim community would support the ME being empowered to issue a burial order, so as to minimise delays. The community are not advocating the power of registration of deaths, but simply the burial order, which is already being issued by deputy registrars for out-of-hours and see no reason why that could not be extended to MEs.

The community is extremely grateful to the National Medical Examiner, Dr Alan Fletcher, for all the hard work that he and his team have done to roll out this new system and for the recent guidance that encourages rapid release of bodies from hospital mortuaries to allow people to bury their loved ones quickly.[3] The community would urge all hospital trusts in the United Kingdom to adopt this guideline so that there is consistency and Table 15.2 lists some of the concerns expressed by the Muslim community that it is believed should be addressed before the MES becomes statutory.

Table 15.2 Concerns expressed by the Muslim community that should be addressed before the Medical Examiner system becomes statutory

1. Out-of-hours	This is crucial for the community and there should be provisions in place at hospitals as well as community practices. The community has encountered delays where the Medical Examiner System has been in place and there were delays in accessing the services of a Medical Examiner. This is probably one of the greatest concerns for the community due to the need to bury their loved ones as quickly as possible. This may become a real issue for community deaths where most GP practices do not have any out-of-hours provision.
2. Delays with the additional layer of paperwork	During the non-statutory phase, contrary to expectations, delays have been very minimal and have not had a negative impact. The Medical Examiner System will need to be adequately resourced so that there is no delay in the process.
3. Independence	There are concerns that if the Medical Examiner System is part of the bereavement office in hospitals this will allow for independence from the Trust in terms of their duties and role. Assurance has been received that their independence will be very much protected, and the National Medical Examiner guidelines will ensure this.
4. Sufficient numbers of Medical Examiners	Given the numbers of Medical Examiners that have undergone training, there is less concern about the availability for the secondary care sector; however, concern remains about the rollout to the primary care sector. The Muslim community does not believe that there are enough Medical Examiners to carry out the new system for all the sectors.
5. Training of staff	It is important that all staff and people involved in the process of death and end-of-life are fully conversant of the requirements of people's faith. The Muslim community is grateful that the current Medical Examiner training includes a portion about faith requirements. However, the community believes this training needs to be extended to all staff who deal with the death and end-of-life process and the community is very happy to work with the sector in order to provide this training.
6. Consistency	With a statutory system in place, it is hoped that there is consistency in delivering this new system by all Medical Examiners. The community has experienced inconsistency in the coronial sector in the level of service provided by different Coroners.
7. Role of National Medical Examiner	We believe that the role should have a legal backing, unlike the current Chief Coroner role, whereby the remit is only on a guidance basis and does not have statutory powers to impose any guidelines. We believe that both roles (National Medical Examiner and Chief Coroner) should have statutory powers in order to ensure that we have consistency and accountability.
8. Charges	For burials, which is the only option for Muslims, there have never been any charges for any certification. We strongly urge that the new system should not introduce any new charges to bereaved families.

In conclusion, the Muslim community, through the National Burial Council, is happy to support the new system, provide any assistance required and share the information about the new statutory system to the wider community.

Hindus and Sikhs

Hindu and Sikh communities do not talk about death until after the event.

If the most densely populated country, India, buried its dead instead of cremating them, there would be no land for the living. In the Hindu scriptures, disposing of human remains is referred to as disintegrating back to nature. It does not stipulate how the body should disintegrate. Traditionally, babies under the age of 2 years and saints are buried. In recent times, babies under 2 years can and have been cremated, subject to the parents' wishes.

In the early years of cremation, the widow was also cremated at the same time as the husband in a practice called Sati. This is now unlawful. Some castes in India still do not permit women in crematoria.

India has fought numerous battles in the past but there is no evidence of the burial of the human remains because those who died were cremated in the battlefields and/or near to where they died, the ashes scattered in a flowing river.

Traditionally in India there is a largely Hindu and Sikh population (see Figure 15.2) and those who have migrated to other parts of the world, with the exception of

Hindu	79.80 %
Muslim	14.23 %
Christian	2.30 %
Sikh	1.72 %
Buddhist	0.70 %
Jain	0.37 %
Other Religion	0.66 %
Not Stated	0.24 %

Figure 15.2   Religious groups in India 2011.[4]

those in the Western world, manage to conclude the cremation ceremony within 24 hours of death.

Upon death, close family members wash the deceased. The final rites are led by the eldest son or daughter; holy water and tulsi herbal leaf are placed in the mouth of the deceased. Mantras are recited; these are messages for the soul to proceed to the next life. The next stage is the cleansing of the residence where the deceased lived, traditionally all bedsheets and a general spring clean.

It is believed that the body should be cremated as soon as possible to give the soul a message that the body it has left is now not in existence after cremation, and subsequently the ashes should be dispersed in a flowing river. It is believed that the soul is present at the time of cremation and until the final prayers of the 13th day.

The next stage of the prayers begins from the 10th day after death with final prayers on the 13th day, which would be the end of the mourning period.

In England there are over 12 000 Hindu and Sikh deaths per annum and while most funerals are concluded within the 13-day mourning period the majority of Hindus and Sikhs conclude the cremation between 5–7 days, which is acceptable.

In order to assist with the ME process, families must be advised to be in touch with the local funeral director so that they are able to simplify the cremation system in place. The community has a concern that when deaths occur at weekends and out of hours, the ME system may cause delays.

Similarly, for unexpected deaths, which may involve the Coroner, the mortuary team and a pathologist, it is important that the bereaved understand the processes involved and how all those involved in the management and support of the bereaved do their utmost to ensure that nothing untoward has happened to their loved one.

Delays in the funeral protocol for the bereaved Hindu or Sikh family can cause a great deal of stress. Clarity of communication, explanation of the process and expected timelines help to minimise the concerns and distress for the families.

Closure for Hindu families is to see their loved one in the coffin and perform the last rites at the deceased's residence. The average attendance at a Hindu funeral is more than 100 mourners. This is part of the Hindu bereavement process to start detaching, by seeing the person dead, and then see the coffin alight, and finally scattering the ashes in the sea or river.

Additionally, Sikh families take the deceased home, then to the temple and then to the crematorium.

Hindus and Sikhs are open-minded about organ donation and post-mortem examinations. Embalming is also permitted to help with the final rite's presentation. Once again distress and concern can be minimised by ensuring good communication.

Judaism

As in all cultures and faiths, the death of a loved one is a time of great intensity and meaning in Jewish families. It is a time to say farewell, mourn and celebrate the life of the deceased. The mourning takes a form that reaffirms the mourners as part of a family, a community and ultimately, a religion. It is a moment when that individual mourner's identity finds expression in their faith tradition in a very profound way. Denial of the ability to express that identity at such a difficult time has the potential to be very damaging for the mourner's mental health. Therefore, it is critical that care for bereaved families is at the heart of the work of NHS trusts and related community care systems, and the post-death legal system in general.

Fulfilling the aims of the MES will provide a service for the common good. The intended systemic improvement in the generation of MCCDs will improve medical learning. The reduction of referrals to Coroners will also support the improvement of coronial performance. However, MEs also serve bereaved families, who are likely to be the initial beneficiaries of (or the first people to be negatively affected by) the work of the ME. As such, the disciplines required for faith-sensitive work – communication, consideration and efficiency – will likely benefit all families whether they have faith or not.

To recognise how to support Jewish families, it should be understood that the keystone of Judaism is a series of covenants, or britot, between God and the Jewish people. These covenants underpin a wide-ranging set of commitments that Jewish people traditionally hold they owe to their God. Those commitments are actualised through mitzvot – biblical commandments understood through the Jewish legal text, the Talmud. As such, the Talmud is the wellspring of Jewish law or halakha. This halakha refers to every facet of life – how to eat, how to work, how to speak and, also, how to mourn. It is important to note that there are differences in levels of observance and approaches to ritual prescription in Jewish communities. Halakha is also sometimes supplemented by traditional practices, which may vary between different observant communities. A traditional Orthodox approach is generally provided here that represents the more ritually prescriptive stream, accepting that even strictly Orthodox-affiliated mourners and families may deviate from or dilute certain practices. The core principles, however, remain.

The actual rituals, customs and traditions performed by Jewish mourners – with notable exceptions – will have very little impact on the work of MEs. But the work of MEs can have a great impact on the Jewish traditions of mourning. If the work of those involved – including the MEs and MEOs – is carried out insensitively it can lead to great distress at such an emotionally vulnerable time. Alternatively, an ME can help ensure that this key phase of someone's life – the loss of a close relative – is lived by the individual as they would wish. It is a profound responsibility.

The two critical elements of Jewish mourning that the work of a ME can impact upon is the timeliness of the funeral, as with other faiths, and ensuring respect for the dead, described in Hebrew as cavod hamet. In practical terms, working towards timely funerals and cavod hamet entails the following:

- The body must not be interfered with. There is an exception to this precept, which is to obey the law of the land. Therefore, post-mortem examinations are allowed when mandated legally. However, every effort should be made to ensure that any interference with the body should be as non-invasive as possible. In the example of post-mortem examinations, imaging and minimal sampling techniques should be used wherever possible.
- If the body is to be interfered with in any way, the family must be consulted to give permission.
- The body must be prepared in a particular way. The preparation – which includes a form of washing – is something the Jewish community has in common with the Muslim community. This is carried out by a Jewish communal organisation called Khevre Kadishe, the 'society of the righteous'. While the body is in the hospital or at home, until it is removed, it is customary that it should not be left alone – traditional Jews who sit with it will often read Tehillim (psalms) while they do so.
- Funerals should take place as soon as possible. Reference guides often say 'within 24 hours' but this is usually stated for ease of reference. In actuality, the halakhic requirement is for the funeral to be held as soon as possible.
- Once the funeral is held, those officially designated as mourners (a mourner is known as an 'ovel', plural 'aveilim') – parents, siblings, spouses and children – follow certain guidelines and restrictions for periods of one week, one month and 12 months after the funeral.

The last point is critical. At the end of the funeral service, the principal mourners, whose outer garments will have had a tear made in them, will walk through the crowd of friends and family, to sit on low chairs. There, the well-wishers will wish them the traditional greeting of 'a long life'. At both the funeral and subsequently, the well-wishers are themselves performing a mitzvah – 'nichum aveilim' – 'comforting the mourners'. The traditional mourning period outlined below cannot commence until the funeral and burial have taken place.

After the funeral, these principal mourners go back to their home for one week, for the 'shiva' period (derived from the Hebrew 'sheva' for seven). Mirrors are covered and doors are left open (at least at specified times), to allow visitors. The mourners do not leave the house. Friends and family visit, particularly at prayer times. The mourners sit on low chairs, and do not wear leather shoes, work, take a full shower or use cosmetics. These traditions – in particular those relating to communal prayer in the house and visitors – were understandably been affected by the COVID-19 pandemic but families did try to adhere to them as closely as possible while remaining safe.

At the end of the week, the mourners 'rise from shiva'. Some restrictions remain in place for 30 days, particularly those regarding listening to music and attending celebrations. These restrictions continue for 12 months for parents and children of the deceased. Children say the memorial kaddish prayer for 11 months after the funeral.

Jewish people – of varying levels of observance of the prescribed rituals – who become mourners will have an expectation of going through this process. They will have visited friends and relations during shiva for their loved ones. Jewish mourners will often say to their rabbi, 'I am not religious, but I want to do this right for my loved one'. It is an act of respect for those who have died. But in addition, the defined process – the knowing how to 'mourn right as Jews'; the knowing they are honouring their loved one; and the managed reintegration of mourners back into the community – is extremely comforting.

Because shiva only begins after the funeral, Jewish mourners describe feeling in an emotional state of 'limbo' before the funeral, particularly when it is delayed, not knowing what to do with themselves or where to go. Not being able to begin the mourning process can be very damaging to their mental wellbeing.

To summarise, following the death of a loved one, Jewish mourners expect a very structured procedure for mourning with dozens of guidelines, and a way forward in terms of re-engaging with the wider community. This process may last for up to one year. This cultural practice is far more structured than that found in general society. It must be made clear to all those handling bereaved families, including MEs and their staff, that the pre-funeral period places the mourner at the other extreme – a sense of loss without any structure whatsoever. The resultant distress can be profound.

Therefore, in general, what Jewish families need from a faith-sensitive post-death legal system is:

- a sense of control, so that they know the body can be cared for by the Khevre Kadishe in the appropriate manner
- not just the expeditious release of the body, but the confidence that it will be expeditiously released.

In practice, both the sense of control, and the confidence that the body will be released will be delegated. When a Jewish loved one dies, usually their family will call the person's synagogue to notify them of the death. They will then contact the burial society and the Khevre Kadishe, who are likely to be the ones that liaise directly with the hospital. Along with the cemetery, these are the critical organisations. Ultimately, the family will want the reassurance that the hospital and these organisations are working well together.

It is vital that MEs build a relationship with whoever leads on burials and support for the bereaved families in their local Jewish community. Indeed, building strong relationships with local faith communities has been identified as an important part of best practice by the National Medical Examiner (NME).[5] Outside London, the community may have a lead person who is associated with the burial society, the Khevre Kadishe or the cemetery. Through the ME's relationship with this lead person, MEs will be able to build a service that supports Jewish families who are mourning. Although there are major concentrations of Jews in cities such as London, Manchester and Leeds, there are Jews and small Jewish communities in many places, so that it is difficult to develop intricate guidelines on how such a service could be delivered. However, any successful system will have the following features:

- In general, there has to be absolute clarity for stakeholders with regards to the geographical jurisdiction of MEs. This is of particular concern as deaths in the community come under the remit of the ME. In theory it should be straightforward to understand how the geographical jurisdiction of the ME relates to NHS jurisdictions and coronial areas. There are concerns within the Jewish community that any confusion may lead to delay, particularly once the system is statutory.
- Death recording should include reference to the faith of the deceased. This exercise would facilitate communication with the Jewish community, and to the Coroner where necessary, as outlined below. The Government's Race Disparity Unit advocated the mandatory recording of ethnicity on death certificates in October 2020, due to the disproportionate mortality impact of COVID-19 on BAME communities.[6] This was echoed in recommendation 2 of the National Medical Examiner's Good Practice Series No. 1, 'How MEs can support people of Black, Asian and minority ethnic heritage and their relatives'.[7] Jews can regard themselves as a minority ethnic group, a faith group, or both, so this proposal will also be of benefit to the Jewish community. The ONS found that, during the first wave of the virus from March to May 2020, Jewish men were more than twice as likely to die from COVID-19 as Christian men, even after a range of socio-economic control factors were taken into account. The Muslim, Hindu and Sikh communities were also disproportionately affected on this measure. The Jewish experience during the pandemic underlines the importance of reporting on Jewish status on death certification so that we can learn from any disproportionalities suffered by the community.

- It should be clear how a family (or their representative) can request early release or prioritisation, as indicated in the good practice guidelines for MEs.[5] The Jewish community appreciates the work undertaken in the National Medical Examiner's Good Practice Series No. 2, 'How MEs can facilitate urgent release of a body', especially the paper's first recommendation, 'Engage positively with local communities that may have particular wishes or needs regarding release of the body'.[3] One test of whether your engagement with faith communities is being successful is whether it is clear to those communities how to request the early release of a body.
- The processing of cases to enable the release of bodies should not be limited to office hours. The NME has already called for an out-of-hours system to be offered as appropriate.[5] Jewish families do not bury their loved ones on the Jewish Sabbath, or Shabbat, which lasts from sunset on Friday evening until Saturday evening or after dark. Therefore, in practice, an out-of-hours service for the Jewish community is needed for early evenings and Sundays.
- All relevant documentation should be retained for scrutiny and follow up, at least until an MCCD has been issued, or a Coroner investigation has been concluded. This will further support the expeditious processing of cases.
- The system should run smoothly and avoid unnecessary delays. The Jewish community advocates that there should be a target of one to three hours for MEs to process MCCDs from the time of notification of a death.
- The family and their representatives should be engaged to ensure post-death rites are respected.
- Examination of the body after death should, wherever possible, be carried out in a non-invasive way, or the least invasive way possible. In the main this requires post-mortem examinations to be carried out using imaging techniques such as CT scans, as opposed to the conventional invasive approach. However, even if digital post mortem is not suitable, invasiveness should be minimised. For example, can post-mortem interference with the body be restricted to skin samples and/or blood samples? And if only samples are required, are there already existing records or samples that can be used?

The number of post-mortem examinations in hospital has radically declined over the last few decades. MEs continue to have a role in minimising the invasiveness of such investigations. However, this is likely to be largely exercised through their communication with Coroners.

Coroners are judicially independent and make any decision regarding what investigations should take place once a case has been referred to them. However, they have traditionally received advice from senior NHS trust staff and GPs on referral, and one can envisage that MEs will also be a useful source of advice.

When referring a case to the Coroner, the Jewish community has suggested the following items are communicated:

- The faith, if any, of the deceased.
- Whether the family requests the swift release of the body. (It should be noted that the High Court upheld the principle that a Coroner can prioritise a case for any suitable reason, including faith considerations, in *R [Adath Yisroel Burial Society)] v Senior Coroner for Inner North London*.[8]
- The maximal invasiveness required for investigations into the cause of death required. For example, can the investigation be completed through the review of pre-existing records? If 'new' evidence needs to be collated, can it be done using imaging techniques? If an invasive investigation must be carried out, can it be limited to samples, for example of skin and blood, rather than a full examination?

The NME has issued guidance regarding communication with faith communities and has been in regular contact with representatives of the Jewish community. The Jewish community appreciates these efforts in regard to those elements of a faith sensitive service that are already included either in Good Practice Guidelines or the Good Practice Series. The Jewish community continue to engage with the NME and his team with regards to issues such as engagement with the families, geographical jurisdiction, recording of faith, expeditious release of bodies, retention of documentation and communication with Coroners.

Conclusions

The role of the ME is intrinsically bound up with care of the deceased and support for the bereaved. Responding to and observing the sensitivities of all faiths, subject to legal needs, must be the aim of all ME services. Progress on issues such as these develops faster when practitioners are generating real-world responses to immediate problems. Learning from such experiences and incorporating this learning into standardised guidance is the best way of progressing. Proactive and continuous communication with all faith communities, adapting to local needs and values is an essential way to improve practice and gives MEs the opportunity to serve these communities in their own area, and advance the MES in the wider multi-ethnic, multifaith and multicultural aspects of society, throughout England and Wales.

REFERENCES

1. Office for National Statistics. 2011 Census. https://www.ons.gov.uk/census/2011census (accessed 20 December 2021).
2. Chief Coroner. Guidance No. 32. Post-Mortem Examinations including Second Post-Mortem Examinations, 2020. https://www.judiciary.uk/wp-content/uploads/2020/08/Guidance-No.-32-Post-Mortem-Examinations-including-Second-Post-Mortem-Examinations-1.pdf (accessed 20 December 2021).

3. The Royal College of Pathologists. National Medical Examiner's Good Practice Series No. 2, 2021. https://www.rcpath.org/uploads/assets/3590bf7f-a43e-4248-980640c5c12354c4/Good-Practice-Series-Urgent-release-of-a-bodyFor-Publication.pdf (accessed 20 December 2021).
4. Census Organization of India. Population Census, 2011. https://www.census2011.co.in/ (accessed 20 December 2021).
5. NHS England. Implementing the Medical Examiner System: National Medical Examiner's Good Practice Guidelines, 2020. https://www.england.nhs.uk/wp-content/uploads/2020/08/National_Medical_Examiner_-_good_practice_guidelines.pdf (accessed 20 December 2021).
6. Public Health England. COVID-19: Review of Disparities in Risks and Outcomes, 2020. https://assets.publishing.service.gov.uk/government/uploads/system/uploads/attachment_data/file/908434/Disparities_in_the_risk_and_outcomes_of_COVID_August_2020_update.pdf (accessed 20 December 2021).
7. The Royal College of Pathologists. National Medical Examiner's National Medical Examiner's Good Practice Series No. 1, 2021. https://www.rcpath.org/uploads/assets/72675084-5ed3-43a1-b518c61395dd1194/Good-Practice-Series-BAME-paper.pdf (accessed 20 December 2021).
8. R (Adath Yisroel Burial Society) v Senior Coroner for Inner North London. EWHC 969, 2018.

CHAPTER 16

The Funeral Director and the Medical Examiner

Brian Parsons

Introduction

In this chapter the relationship between the funeral director and Medical Examiner (ME) is explored. Caring for the deceased person is but one task of the funeral director. It is, however, a primary one as no funeral can take place without a body. Funeral directors transfer the deceased from the place of death into their custody and give advice to the bereaved about certification and death registration. It is in this capacity that the funeral director may well interact with the ME.

The first part of this chapter examines the function of the funeral director. The next section focuses on the current system of death and certification and management of the deceased person. The final paragraphs discuss the implications of broadening the Medical Examiner role to include deaths in the community.

What do funeral directors do?

Funeral directors arrange and direct funerals in addition to providing care for the deceased in the interval between death and the funeral. The role is as much about caring for the living as for the deceased. The funeral director must always be available in time of need and be capable of providing practical support along with expert help and advice. The noted American writer on death and bereavement, Rabbi Earl A Grollman, described the funeral director as:

> ... *Caretaker, caregiver and gatekeeper; that is caretaker of the dead, caregiver to the bereaved... [and]... from the perspective of the community... the secular gatekeeper between the living and the dead.* (Quoted in Leming and Dickinson 1985: 467.[1])

DOI: 10.1201/9781003188759-16

The characteristics of a funeral director can be listed as:

- *Master of ceremonies*: guiding the family during the time of the funeral. Funerals vary from the simple to the complex, requiring planning, logistical input concerning transport and staff, and negotiations with third parties (see below). Attention to detail and a problem-solving approach are essential characteristics of a funeral director.
- *Custodian of the dead*: transporting and providing care of the body in a climate-controlled environment, and also access to the body in a viewing facility. Arterial embalming is offered by many funeral directors to provide temporary preservation of the deceased.
- *Contractor*: when a client arranges a funeral the funeral director becomes responsible for providing goods, services and facilities as negotiated. In return the client has an obligation to settle the account. Funeral directors operate in a confidential environment and can only disclose details to the appointed client, although as Conway notes, establishing who is entitled to make funeral arrangements is not entirely clear and conflict concerning decisions are not unknown to funeral directors.[2]
- *Technical advisor*: giving information to the client on matters concerning the registration of death, Coroner's procedure, burial and cremation legislation, international transportation of remains, exhumation and options concerning ceremonial matters, etc.
- *Agent*: depending upon the arrangements, the funeral director is required to liaise with the following: the registrar of deaths, the Coroner, doctors, hospital patients' affairs, cemeteries and crematoria, religious and non-religious officiants, monumental masons, airlines, embassy and consular authorities, newspapers, florists, printers, musicians, etc. The Medical Examiner can be added to this list.

Table 16.1   Activities a funeral directing business must be able to undertake

- Arranging, administering and directing instructions received for cremations and burials along with the international transportation of human remains and ashes
- Providing a range of coffins and caskets along with urns for ashes and other items such as a temporary grave marker
- A 24-hour telephone response to all enquiries
- Conveying the deceased from the place of death to the funeral director's mortuary on the instructions of a client or third party such as such as a Coroner, hospital trust, Network Rail, etc.
- Preparation of the deceased for viewing, which may include arterial embalming
- The removal of pacemakers or other implants from the deceased
- The transportation of the coffin and also ashes throughout the UK and internationally
- The receiving of the deceased from outside the UK and arranging local burial or cremation
- Children's funerals, including non-viable fetuses
- Managing double and multiple funerals
- Arranging the burial and cremation of body parts
- Contracting with local and health authorities to arrange funerals under section 46 of the Public Health (Control of Disease) Act 1984
- Arranging direct (non-attended) cremations
- Arranging the bequeathal of a body for anatomical dissection and carrying out the funeral at a later date
- Arranging the exhumation of human remains and ashes, along with facilitating reburial, transportation or cremation
- Offering a range of pre-need/pre-paid funeral plans
- Providing monumental masonry services, including new memorials, removing and replacing the memorial for reopening a grave and for renovation work, including adding an inscription

The Funeral Industry

The Competition and Markets Authorities report (2020) estimates that in 2017 there were 6995 funeral directing businesses (including branches of large organisations) in the UK.[3] The estimated market share is as follows: the Co-operative Group (not including regional societies) 17%, Dignity PLC 13% and Funeral Partners 3%, with the remaining 67% in the hands of the independent/family sector.

There are two main trade associations that funeral directors can join, although this is not mandatory. The National Association of Funeral Directors (NAFD) was founded in 1905 and represents over 4100 funeral directors, while the National Society of Allied and Independent Funeral Directors (SAIF) provides membership for firms not owned by nationwide companies. There is a proposed joint Code of Practice.[4] The vast majority of funerals are arranged through a funeral director, although there is no requirement to use one.

Death and Contact with the Funeral Director

When a death occurs (and sometimes before), contact is made with the funeral director to discuss funeral arrangements and take custody of a deceased. Advice on the registration of death or the involvement of the Coroner will be offered, followed by a conversation to gather information about the deceased, the client, the place of burial or cremation, format of service and details such as music, flowers, donations, transport, death notices or an online announcement, and disposition of ashes. Further discussion concerning care and treatment of the deceased will include whether embalming is to take place, viewing, dressing, removal of implants, jewellery and personal effects. The funeral director will also offer a range of coffins, book a date and time for the funeral and provide an estimate of costs. A summary of the activities that will need to be undertaken by the funeral director is shown in Table 16.1.

Death and Certification

Irrespective of where death occurs, a decision will have to be taken about whether a referral needs to be made to the Coroner in whose jurisdiction the person is lying. This will depend on the circumstances, if the cause of death is known, whether the Registered Medical Practitioner (RMP – doctor) has seen the person alive during the appointed timeframe prior to death, and/or whether there is a legal requirement, such as death in state detention. If the death is not referred, a Medical Certificate of Cause of Death (MCCD) will be issued by the doctor. It may also be supplied if a referral is made to the Coroner, but after discussion there is no intervention. The MCCD is transmitted to the Registrar, usually by email, and the informant is required to register within five days of the date of death. It is possible for the informant to delay the registration by notifying the registrar and submitting the MCCD, then returning at a later date to carry out full registration. Upon notification, the registrar can issue the Certificate for Burial and Cremation. This opportunity to delay the registration but hold the funeral is particularly helpful for faiths that require prompt burial or cremation.

Delays in issuing the MCCD can be caused by the workload of the RMP and/or their availability. If the only doctor who can complete this document is absent, for example due to illness or holiday, then this document cannot be issued and the death cannot be registered.

Deaths in Hospitals

The majority of deaths occur in hospitals and nursing homes; in 2016 it was 46.9% and 21.8% respectively. There is, however, a trend towards a reduction of hospital deaths; in 2004 it was 57.9%.[5] The body will be removed from the ward to the mortuary to be kept in a climate-controlled environment. In some circumstances the body will be removed to a Coroner's mortuary for a post-mortem examination, although sometimes this may be the same location. The bereavement office will provide a release document to the next to kin, which is then passed to the funeral director (see Chapter 8). The mortuary will require this signed authority before the body is released; in cases where this document is not provided, the mortuary will need sight of the registrar's Certificate for Burial and Cremation to prove the funeral director's entitlement to custody of the body (see Chapter 17). The body will only be released after the MCCD has been completed. In the case of cremation, only the Medical Certificate (Cremation Form 4) is required.

Embalming and Preparation of the Deceased

Many funeral directors offer embalming. The treatment involves injection through an artery (such as the right common carotid, or right or left femoral) using a formaldehyde-based fluid and then withdrawing the blood from the right auricle using a hollow needle (a trocar). On occasion more than one artery is selected, particularly if a thorough saturation of the tissue is required such as if the body is being transported abroad or there is a delay until the funeral. When injection is complete a strong fluid is injected into the abdominal and thoracic cavities. The mouth and eyes are closed, the hair is groomed and if the deceased is male he is shaved.

If the body is subject to a post-mortem examination, the chest cavity and head are reopened, and the soft organs are removed and sanitised. Arteries in the neck, arms and legs are then individually injected. The organs are replaced, the cavity is re-sutured and the body is externally cleansed. Facial features are set and cosmetics applied according to need.

Embalming effectively prevents deterioration of the body in the interval between death and the funeral. This is particularly important if the deceased is to be dressed in their own clothing and/or there is a delay prior to the funeral. If a deceased is to be transported abroad, then either airlines or consular authorities usually stipulate that thorough embalming is carried out. Embalming improves presentation of the deceased through giving a more natural skin colour. Injection and massage of the skin can also remove post-mortem staining, particularly if this has occurred in the face. In the case of a body subjected to a post-mortem examination, embalming can prevent leakage from the stitching to the head and cavity.

Although retaining the body in climate-controlled conditions achieves preservation, it does not address presentational aspects. In addition, many funeral directors do not have refrigeration at all their premises; bodies will often be embalmed in a central mortuary and transferred to the viewing facility where they will remain until the funeral.

Before embalming can take place, the death must be registered/notified and Cremation Form 4 issued. If the death has been reported to the Coroner, then one of the following will be issued: the registrar's Certificate for Burial; a Coroner's Burial Order (Form 101); or the Coroner's Certificate for Cremation (Cremation Form 6). The client must also have agreed either verbally or in writing to the deceased being embalmed. If a deceased is to be transported abroad a certificate needs to be signed by the embalmer. The British Institute of Embalmers provides a system for training and qualification, although there is no prerequisite for embalmers to be qualified before practising.[6]

The Funeral Director and Coronavirus

The Coronavirus Act 2020 resulted in a number of changes affecting funeral directors: the registration of death by telephone, including the opportunity for the funeral director to act as informant; the suspension of the Confirmatory Medical Certificate (Cremation Form 5); an increase from 14 to 28 days for the time in which a doctor must have seen the person alive before completing the MCCD; electronic transfer of the MCCD along with certificates for burial and cremation to cemeteries and crematoria; and restrictions on the number of mourners attending funerals.[7] In the absence of nationwide operational directives and influenced by the volume of funerals being managed, funeral directors adopted their own policies regarding their service provision on matters such as limousines, the range of coffins, withdrawing embalming and not permitting viewing of COVID-19 cases. In addition, cremation and burial authorities amended their arrangements on matters including the length of service in a crematorium, capacity in the chapel and their insistence that the coffin is lowered immediately upon arrival at the grave.[8]

In preparation for an excess number of deaths, some local authorities arranged for 'overflow' mortuaries to be constructed to which the deceased could be moved, pending collection by the funeral director. The transfer between a hospital or Coroner's mortuary to such a mortuary would be carried out by a funeral director on the instructions of local authority or hospitals. Some funeral directors also had temporary mortuary facilities.

The Coronavirus Act received royal assent on 25 March 2020 and required renewal every six months until it expired on 24th March 2022. Since this legislation expired, certain provisions are continuing; that the RMP must have seen the person during the last 28 days (not 14); the MCCD can be submitted electronically to the registrar; Cremation Form 5 has been permanently removed.

The Funeral Director and the Medical Examiner

The introduction of the Medical Examiner system, including the pilot schemes, have been well covered in funeral-directing periodicals and on conference agendas over a number of years. Anecdotal information from funeral directors who deal with hospitals where the system is in operation reported very few issues arising from such matters as delays in supply of the MCCD and/or release of the body. As discussion regarding the MCCD is regarded as an internal matter between professionals in the hospital, there is little need for involvement of the funeral director. It may, however, be the case that the next of kin ask the funeral director about how the system operates. For this reason, the funeral director must be able to contact the ME Service, and also in circumstances when problems with certification occur.

Widening the remit of the Medical Examiner system to include deaths in the community raises a number of issues. The first concerns who can verify a death. Previously this was discussed in the Brodrick Report (1971)[9] and also Deaths in the Community (1986).[10] The BMA's current guidance states that doctors are under no legal obligation to attend a home or nursing facility to confirm an expected death.[11] The extinction of life can be verified by a 'competent person', which in practice includes a general practitioner, locum doctor, paramedic or senior nursing home member of staff. The degree of prior clinical experience to carry out this task, however, is not specified. What is certain is that funeral directors and embalmers should not be requested to do this as they are not trained in verification techniques; their function is dealing with the dead, not the 'possibly' or 'thought to be' dead. Only when a funeral director has received notification of death at a home or nursing facility and knows that verification has taken place should transfer of the deceased into their care take place.

A second issue concerns the potential for delay where faith requirements stipulate that burial or cremation takes place within a short timeframe. Following death in the community and subsequent verification, the doctor in attendance during the last illness must complete the MCCD for forwarding to the Medical Examiner service. If this RMP is unavailable and/or there is no Medical Examiner available to scrutinise the MCCD, death cannot be registered and no funeral can take place. Suitable arrangements must be in place to ensure that another doctor can complete the MCCD and that there is adequate out-of-hours access to a Medical Examiner. In situations where a delay is encountered it usually results in the funeral director having to explain the reasons to the family and also attempting to expedite the process. Furthermore, the deceased must remain in appropriate surroundings in the custody of the funeral director, a situation that may well have an impact on funeral costs.

Lastly, the issue of whether a client needs to pay for the MES once the system becomes statutory needs clarification, particularly if it is expected that the funeral director is to collect a fee. Although funeral directors regularly obtain disbursements from their clients for third party expenses (and often before the funeral takes place) – such as the cremation fee, Cremation Form 4, and purchase of and interment in a grave – the mechanism for receipting and distributing the charge needs to be brought to the attention of all funeral directors before the system is commenced.

Overall, the funeral directing community supports the Medical Examiner system as it attempts to reassure the newly bereaved concerning the cause of death.

REFERENCES

1. Leming MR, Dickinson GE. *Understanding Death, Dying and Bereavement*, 3e. New York: Holt McDougal; 1985.
2. Conway H. *The Law and the Dead*. Oxford: Routledge; 2018.
3. Competition and Markets Authority. Funerals Market Investigation Final Report, 2020 https://assets.publishing.service.gov.uk/media/5fdb557e8fa8f54d5733f5a1/Funerals_-_Final_report.pdf (Accessed 3 April 2021)
4. National Association of Funeral Directors (NAFD). The Funeral Director Code. https://www.nafd.org.uk/standards/the-funeral-director-code/?msclkid=9527aa80af7c11ec8a8b8d20c44f bdb7 (Accessed 3 April 2021)
5. GOV.uk. Statistical commentary: End of Life Care Profiles, 2018. https://www.gov.uk/government/statistics/end-of-life-care-profiles-february-2018-update/statistical-commentary-end-of-life-care-profiles-february-2018-update#main-findings (accessed 20 December 2021).
6. British Institute of Embalmers. www.bioe.co.uk (accessed 20 December 2021).
7. GOV.uk. Coronavirus Act, 2020. https://www.legislation.gov.uk/ukpga/2020/7/enacted (accessed 20 December 2021).
8. Mortlake Crematorium. Covid, 2021. https://www.mortlakecrematorium.org/coronavirus/ (accessed 20 December 2021).
9. Report of the Committee on Death Certification and Coroners, London, 1971.
10. Deaths in the Community. London: British Medical Association (1986)
11. British Medical Association. Verification of Death (VoD), 2020. https://www.bma.org.uk/media/2843/bma-verification-of-death-vod-july-2020.pdf (accessed 20 December 2021).

CHAPTER 17

The Role of the Mortuary

Lee Gibbs and John Pitchers

Introduction

The English dictionary defines a mortuary as *'a building or a room in a hospital where dead bodies are kept before they are buried or cremated, or before they are identified or examined'*. In the United States a mortuary has been defined as follows: *'A mortuary is the same as a funeral home'*.

A modern mortuary facility embraces both of these descriptions and more.

This chapter will explore general, UK mortuary services using national guidelines, information from governing bodies and the personal experiences of senior mortuary anatomical pathology technologists (APT) operating in the Norfolk and Norwich University Hospital NHS Foundation Trust mortuary, the sixth largest mortuary in the UK.

How Mortuaries Were Established

Historically, mortuaries were set up as a means to counter the appalling conditions that surrounded death processes. In heavily populated areas of London, for example, burial grounds were limited and often so short of space that the deceased were regularly buried just inches below the ground.

Relatives of the deceased were often expected to keep the bodies of their loved ones in their dwelling for long periods of time, during which decomposition of the body would occur. Often the deceased would have been kept in the same room as others going about their daily business. In 1854, the Westminster coroner expressed his disgust to St Anne's burial board at having been compelled, with his jury, to view a body 'in a far advanced state of decomposition' lying in a house containing 20 residents.[1]

The Public Health Act of 1848 enabled the London local boards of health to provide mortuaries. The first London parish to provide a mortuary was St Anne, Soho. Limited mortuary facilities, known as 'dead-houses', were also available within institutions, such as hospitals, prisons, asylums and workhouses, for the short-term storage of those who had died there. Other bodies might be taken there by agreement, such as in 1867, when the master of the St Marylebone workhouse agreed to receive the bodies of some 40 skaters who had died when the ice on a lake in Regent's Park suddenly gave way.

Looking after a deceased person at home at that time was considered to be the normal and decent thing to do. Regular mortuaries, as we know them today, would not be commonplace until well into the twentieth century.

Modern Mortuaries

The size of modern mortuaries is usually determined by local authorities and hospitals, taking into account historic data about coroners' caseloads and hospital mortuary usage, as well as projected future requirements. All trusts record their own data around mortality and feed into a national mortality register that provides details to central government and allows these council districts to make those decisions on the provision of mortuary space. All mortuaries have contingency plans for when demand outstrips capacity, such as during the winter months. Additional arrangements have had to be made during the coronavirus pandemic, with existing mortuaries being expanded and temporary mortuaries being established.

Norfolk is one of the largest coroner areas in the UK, with coronial post-mortem examinations distributed across three large acute hospital-based mortuaries. London, in comparison, is split into many districts with numerous smaller public and hospital mortuaries.

Public mortuaries

Public mortuaries are 'stand-alone', meaning they are operated by a local authority on behalf of the coroner and are not attached to a hospital or other similar facility. They generally consist of storage for deceased patients who have died within the coroner's area, and post-mortem and viewing/formal ID facilities. These mortuaries may care for patients who have died in the community or in hospitals with no post-mortem facilities.

Hospital mortuaries

Hospital mortuaries are NHS-operated facilities, handling in-patient deaths. Some hospital mortuaries also undertake public mortuary duties for the surrounding community and coroner, where there is no stand-alone public mortuary.

The Norfolk and Norwich University Hospital NHS Foundation Trust (NNUH) mortuary, for example, is the sixth largest in the country with 104 permanent refrigerated spaces and handles 3800–4200 deceased patients annually. Of these, approximately 2500 deaths take place within the hospital. The mortuary serves the hospital in all aspects including storage, viewing/identification processes and hospital/consented post-mortem examinations where requested.

The mortuary also serves the Norfolk coroner, whose jurisdiction embraces around 1.2 million people. The mortuary undertakes between 850 and 1150 post-mortem examinations per year.

Staffing

Almost all mortuaries and their services are run and managed by anatomical pathology technologists (APTs), many of whom enter the profession from allied services such as nursing, care work, laboratory work or funeral services. The APT role is a highly specialised one within the life sciences strand of the health-care science workforce, and APT staff require upwards of three or four years of on-the-job technical training and academic study to be able to practice independently.[2] Ultimately the APT's main role is to ensure the deceased is treated with care, understanding and empathy throughout the mortuary and post-mortem process.

The APT qualifications have changed in status and style over the last 10 years. Currently, Level 3 and 4 Diplomas in Anatomical Pathology Technology are awarded, with training and certification being provided by the Royal Society of Public Health (RSPH) alongside the APT's governing body, the Association of Anatomical Pathology Technology (AAPT). Some senior mortuary staff hold additional qualifications such as embalming, counselling or specialist reconstructive skills, which aid their departments in caring for those patients that may have died in traumatic ways, and their relatives.

APTs work alongside histopathologists, the majority of whom also undertake diagnostic surgical pathology. These doctors are qualified to perform post-mortem examinations to establish the cause of death. Mortuaries require a licence from the Human Tissue Authority (HTA)[3] in order to carry out post-mortems legally, in addition to many other licensable activities. Many APTs assist by performing post-mortem evisceration (removal of the deceased patient's organs and tissues) under the supervision of a histopathologist. The histopathologist will then dissect the tissues further, examine and weigh the organs, and hopefully establish the cause of death.

Home Office-registered forensic pathologists are tasked with carrying out post-mortem examinations on cases that are potentially criminal, such as homicide, manslaughter or certain road traffic offences. These cases are ordered by the coroner after formal police investigation and the attendance of crime scene investigators.

Some mortuaries also employ mortuary assistants to aid in manual handling and ancillary work. Some also employ staff in administrative roles to assist with the ever-increasing amount of data collection and input.

All of these staff come together to provide a full and varied mortuary service to both internal and external stakeholders. In terms of process, it can loosely be described as outlined below.

Admission and Storage of Deceased Patients

Hospital and public mortuaries are required to admit and store deceased patients and their personal effects safely and securely. On admission, an administrative process will be completed to show where the deceased is, what identifying details they possess, and what personal effects they have on or about their person. Most mortuaries will be required to add an additional, unique identifying number that follows the patient whenever they are moved or examined and checks on that location are expected to be performed throughout to maintain safety and continuity.

Deceased patients may be admitted from a number of places. Hospital mortuaries will accept inpatient deaths on a 24/7 basis, with most using independent or trust portering services in and out of hours. Any hospital or public mortuary that deals with coroners' cases will also usually accept community deaths on the same basis, either by providing an on call APT, portering services or other agreed allied professional service to accept patients out of normal office hours. Deceased patients from the community are generally collected from their place of death and delivered to mortuaries by funeral directors who hold a contract with the local coroner or local authority to provide that service. Deceased patients may also be delivered by emergency ambulance should the death have occurred in a public place, or by British Transport Police if it occurred in a train station or on a railway line. Forensic cases are usually admitted to mortuaries at an agreed time with police or a major investigation team officer escort to maintain continuity of the case.

Mortuaries are required to provide body storage spaces of suitable size, width, temperature and security to facilitate safe, secure storage of the deceased. Patients are, of course, different sizes, heights and weights, and arrive at the mortuary in differing conditions. Accurate identification of the body and its location is of paramount importance. Deceased patients can be kept in refrigerated storage for up to 30 days at normal fridge temperatures (around 5°c), after which the Human Tissue Authority recommends moving the body to deep freeze storage for longer periods, to prevent further deterioration of the body. Deep freeze temperatures are around −18°C and the deceased can be kept at this temperature for an indefinite period as required. Some cases can require storage periods of many months dependent on the history. Forensic cases may be kept for longer periods due to the complexities of the examination, processing time of criminal evidence and time to build criminal cases.

Natural or Non-Coronial Death

Hospital inpatients whose death is thought to be natural will still be formally reviewed. Whether the bereaved's next of kin requests a burial or cremation, paperwork will still need to be created and the death will require scrutiny by the Medical Examiner Service, which may include conversations with the deceased's GP and/or the hospital clinical team who treated them at the end of their life. If a natural death can be confirmed following these conversations, then the MCCD is completed, and the death registered with the local register office. Once registered, the deceased can be collected by the family's chosen funeral director.

Hospital or Consented Post-Mortem

Hospital patients dying a natural death can have a post-mortem examination requested by the clinical team, but it will only be completed upon gaining full and informed consent from the family. These are called hospital or consented post-mortems and a member of the family (fulfilling an agreed qualifying relationship to the deceased under HTA regulations) can provide consent to either a full or limited post-mortem examination. A limited post-mortem may confine the examination to the chest or abdomen, for example, or be limited to a tissue biopsy. The family can refuse the request as it is not part of any legal requirement to establish the cause of death.

Hospital post-mortems are usually requested by clinical teams to investigate the route of spread or extent of disease, the response to treatment, or if the disease is rare and learning can be had from investigating further. There may also be a hospital PM request if the deceased may have had a disease with a genetic component so that the risk to surviving family members can be assessed and steps taken to reduce their risk of dying from the same condition.

In Norwich, the family is initially called by the patient's consultant to discuss the possibility of a hospital post-mortem examination. If they agree to attend to discuss the consent, a 'consent trained' member of the mortuary team or other qualified person explains the process, completes the consent form and answers any questions or concerns the family may have. The duty of the person taking consent is to provide full and frank information to the bereaved family on which they can make an informed choice, not to influence their decision about whether or not to give consent. The family are also able to limit the examination to any specific part of the body or specific tissues with limited invasive processes as they wish. After giving consent, the family are given the opportunity to change their mind by means of a cooling off period in which the examination request can be halted. Families are often concerned that a post-mortem examination will delay funeral arrangements, but this is rarely the case. Families can give consent for the retention of tissue for diagnosis, research or teaching.

Coronial Death or Coroner's Referral

Establishing the cause of death is not always easy. The deceased may not have been recently treated or seen by their general practitioner (GP) or other clinicians, as is often the case with the elderly. The GP or hospital clinician also may not have treated the patient long enough or feel confident enough to sign the medical certificate of the cause of death with a natural cause. A range of other circumstances compel notification to the coroner (see Chapters 3 and 10) and are equally applicable in the community and in acute NHS trusts and health boards.

In the community setting, any death that occurs in a deceased person's home, care setting or public place will require the police to attend to complete a sudden death report. This report will usually include the name, address, place of death, next of kin details and some information about how the deceased was found, when and where the body was placed, and so on. This information is then often sent via secure email to the coroner's office where the coroner's officers will investigate and scrutinise the case. They will attempt to contact close family members if they are identified, as well as the patient's GP, to determine any underlying illnesses that may result in a natural cause in the first instance. If no natural cause can be established, the coroner will order a post-mortem examination. Paperwork signed by the coroner to request the post-mortem will be created by the coroner's office and sent to the assigned mortuary via secure email. This document acts as authority for mortuary teams to facilitate and perform the post-mortem examination.

Most mortuaries within coroners' areas will have their own standard operating procedures. For example, some coroners require that, if coronial consent for the bereaved to view or identify the deceased prior to post-mortem has been given, the patient's body must not be disrupted/tampered with, and the family are not permitted to touch the deceased. This may be for forensic and evidential reasons, but can potentially cause the bereaved additional distress, as the mortuary is not able to clean and prepare the deceased for viewing. The family may have been in attendance as the deceased died and they often struggle to understand why they are no longer allowed to touch them once they are in the care of the mortuary. This highlights the importance of having trained and empathetic staff who understand and can explain why there may be certain restrictions in place during a viewing or identification. Coroners vary in their requirements.

Coroner's Post-Mortem Examination

Once authorisation from the coroner is received, the post-mortem is scheduled, and the relevant information is passed to the assigned histopathologist. This usually occurs within one working day of receipt. The deceased will be fully examined externally and internally by the pathologist, supported by APT staff, who will also fully reconstruct the deceased afterwards. Dependent on the condition of the body on its arrival, the body will remain viewable after examination and reconstruction in almost all cases.

The coroner's post-mortem is different from a hospital post-mortem in the sense that a coroner's post-mortem is a requirement of law and not by consent of the family. In a coroner case, the family cannot refuse a post-mortem without significant reason to do so. It is also unlikely for a coroner's post-mortem to be limited to any one organ or part of the body in the same way a hospital post-mortem can be, unless the coroner has given express permission. Most coroner's post-mortems are 'full' examinations requiring examination of all organs and the body as a whole.

The coroner has jurisdiction over the deceased at this stage and may give authority to the histopathologist to retain any organ, tissue or part of the body for the purposes of establishing the cause of death or the identity of the deceased.

The Human Tissue Act 2004 and the Human Tissue Authority

The Human Tissue Authority (HTA) is a regulator set up in 2005 following events in the 1990s that revealed a culture in some hospitals of removing and retaining human organs and tissue without consent. Public inquiries including an inquiry into children's heart surgery at the Bristol Royal Infirmary (BRI) in 2001[4] and the Royal Liverpool Children's Inquiry[5] discovered that organs and tissues had been collected and retained from deceased babies and children for undisclosed periods without the consent of the next of kin. The HTA was established by the Human Tissue Act 2004 (the Act)[6]. The HTA license and inspect organisations that remove, store and use human tissue for research, medical treatment, post-mortem examination, education and training, and display in public. The HTA also endeavours to ensure organ and stem cell donations from living people for the purpose of transplantation do not involve any reward or coercion[6, 7]. The HTAs core functions are set out in the Act and three other pieces of legislation:

- the Human Tissue (Quality and Safety for Human Application) Regulations 2007
- the Quality and Safety of Organs Intended for Transplantation Regulations 2012
- the Human Transplantation (Wales) Act 2013.

These laws are intended to ensure human tissue is used safely and ethically, with appropriate consent.

The Act covers England, Wales and Northern Ireland. The Regulations listed above set out the legal requirements for England, Scotland, Wales and Northern Ireland for the sectors to which they apply (human application and organ donations and transplantation). The Human Transplantation (Wales) Act 2013 sets out the framework for deceased organ donation in Wales.

The Act requires that appropriate consent be in place. The nature of that consent varies depending on the purpose (referred to as a scheduled purpose). There are different consent requirements for some purposes depending on whether with the tissue is from the deceased or the living. Table 17.1 shows those purposes when consent is required, whether the person is alive or dead at the time the material is collected or removed.

There are certain scheduled purposes that require consent for tissue or organs taken from the deceased but *not* from the living. In order to carry out any of the activities listed in Table 17.2 with tissue collected or removed from the deceased, appropriate consent must have been given. However if a person dies after the tissue is taken, it can still be used for these activities without their consent having been taken.

In the case of public display and anatomical examination, removal cannot take place based on someone else's consent; if consent was not obtained from the individual before they died, the tissue or organ(s) cannot be taken. For all other cases listed above, consent can be obtained from someone else who has a 'qualifying relationship'. Table 17.3 identifies the 'qualifying relationships', which are ranked in order.

Each licensed premises is required to have a licence holder (often a senior hospital or divisional manager) with overall legal responsibility, and a designated individual (DI), often a histopathologist or laboratory lead, responsible for ensuring that key staff are trained appropriately, and suitable processes are in place. Lastly,

---

Table 17.1   Consent for the following purposes is required whether the person is alive or dead at the time the material is removed

- Anatomical examination: the use of a body, body part or tissue to teach students or healthcare professionals about the functioning of the human body
- Determining the cause of death: carrying out a post-mortem examination of a body to find out how a person died
- Establishing after a person's death the efficacy of any drug or other treatment administered to them: carrying out tests on cells, tissues, organs or tissue from a deceased person to investigate whether specific treatments they had were effective
- Obtaining scientific or medical information about a living or deceased person which may be relevant to any other person (including a future person): carrying out tests on cells, tissue or organs or tissue from a living or deceased person to find out whether they had any unknown medical or genetic disorders
- Public display: showing a body, body part or tissue to members of the public
- Research in connection with disorders, or the functioning, of the human body: the use of cells, tissues or organs to find out more about how the body and/or disease work
- Transplantation: the removal of an organ or tissue from one person for implanting into another person

Source: Adapted from the Human Tissue Act 2004: A Guide for the Public.

Table 17.2   Scheduled purposes where consent is required for tissue or organs taken from the deceased but not from the living

- Clinical audit: the review of processes used to test tissue, to check whether the right tests have been carried out and whether they have been carried out correctly
- Education or training relating to human health: the use of human tissue to train students and healthcare or medical professionals
- Performance assessment: using human tissue to evaluate and assess diagnostic kits or medical devices
- Public health monitoring: using human tissue to identify and observe health or disease trends in the general public or specific groups
- Quality assurance: the use of tissue to monitor and evaluate a particular research project or health service to make sure effective clinical procedures and diagnostic tests are being used

Source: Adapted from the Human Tissue Act 2004: A Guide for the Public.

Table 17.3 Ranked qualifying relationships for the purpose of consent

1. Spouse or partner (including civil or same sex partner)*
2. Parent or child
3. Brother or sister
4. Grandparent or grandchild
5. Niece or nephew
6. Stepfather or stepmother
7. Half-brother or half-sister
8. Friend of long standing

* For these purposes, a person is considered a partner if they live as partners in an enduring family relationship.
Source: Adapted from the Human Tissue Act 2004: A Guide for the Public.

persons designate (PDs) are appointed to ensure the safe and ethical day-to-day processes relating to relevant materials. Licensed premises are required to hold specific licenses for each outlined scheduled purpose they fulfil and are required to ensure that they comply with all regulations relating to that license. The HTA can also inspect documentation, premises and processes at any time. Prison sentences, heavy fines, closure of services and other restrictive measures can be imposed if licensed services do not comply with HTA regulations.

Retention of tissue

Sometimes the cause of death cannot be established macroscopically during the post-mortem examination and the histopathologist may need to retain whole organs or small pieces of tissue to examine under a microscope. The coroner still holds jurisdiction and responsibility for these organs and/or tissues until such time as the cause of death is established. At that point the jurisdiction and responsibility for the outstanding tissues or organs reverts back to the next of kin and it is they who must decide what happens to those tissues once the examination is completed. The pathologist informs the coroner of any tissue retained following every post-mortem examination. The coroner will send a consent form to the next of kin so they can outline their wishes for how they wish for any retained organs or tissues to be disposed of.

They have five options (the first three being statutory) open to them:

- Return the tissues to the body before the funeral (delay release of the body to a funeral director until such time as the tissues can be repatriated to the deceased)
- Retain the tissues as part of the medical record (hold the material in a biorepository for a period of 30 years as part of the deceased person's medical record at which time the tissues will be incinerated as clinical waste)
- Retain the tissues as part of the medical record and use them in ethically approved research (hold the material in a biorepository for a period of 30 years as part of the deceased person's medical record and make them

available for ethically approved research bodies for that period, at which time the tissues will be incinerated as clinical waste)

- Hospital disposal (clinical incineration after the tissues have been used for their scheduled purpose)
- Return to me (return the tissues to the designated next of kin, sometimes even after the funeral. The tissues will be delivered in a safe condition to handle).

In the mortuary setting, it is the responsibility of the person/s designate (PD/s) to ensure that the wishes of the next of kin are fulfilled and the tissues are handled in accordance with the consent and the law. The process is documented against the patient's admission record at each step. Processes are also in place to ensure that deceased patients are not released to funeral agencies without the appropriate documented procedures first taking place.

Organ donation

Organ donation can occur in a number of ways. Consent to donate organs is obviously paramount and is, again, regulated under the HTA licence for each trust that performs them. Consent is usually obtained from the deceased's next of kin by a specialist nurse – organ donation (SNOD) team in an acute trust setting. The donation or retrieval of organs is generally performed in a hospital operating theatre at the point of legally recognised death. The donor may be heart-beating but clinically 'brainstem' deceased or ventilated, and clinically deceased. In such cases, whole organs such as the heart, lungs and liver may be retrieved for transplantation. If the cause of death is deemed to be unnatural, the coroner will also have to give consent for any retrieval based on the possibility of loss of pathology or findings at any subsequent post-mortem required.

Organ donation that is less time-specific can take place in the mortuary following a longer interval after death. The organs and tissues that donors can consent to donating in the mortuary include heart valves, skin, bone, tendons, eye and other research tissues. These can be collected up to 24 hours after death and are usually retrieved by specialist organ donation teams that visit the mortuary.[6] Mortuary APT staff assist in some cases and some hold qualifications or have experience in enucleation (eye/ocular retrieval), for example. The deceased is reconstructed fully after any retrieval so that they remain viewable by the next of kin without any visible external disruption.

Viewing and Identification of Deceased Patients

Most mortuaries, either public or hospital, will have the means to facilitate viewing and identification of the deceased. The NNUH mortuary, for example, performs 850–1000 viewings and identifications annually. Most mortuaries have a dedicated viewing room or bereavement suite. These usually feature a religion-neutral space in which the deceased can be presented in a natural and sensitive fashion and where bereaved people can spend time with their loved one. The family can be supported throughout their viewing as required by trained APT staff. APT staff take pride in their ability to support the bereaved during such difficult times and to be there to answer any question or allay any fears or concerns the visitors may have.

The same will apply for police/coroner identification, in which the only difference is that the identification is a legal process and is formally documented. The identification is often jointly conducted by an APT and a police or coroner's officer to fulfil the completion of identification documents for the coroner. The coroner will require formal ID to be able to open an inquest on any death requiring an inquest, such as a fall or road traffic collision. The nominated bereaved person will provide a positive ID to the attending police officer and sign a witness statement to confirm that fact. The ID statement will form part of the deceased patient's record for post-mortem, and so on. Formal ID can occur after post-mortem examination if necessary.

Release of the Deceased

Once a post-mortem and all other investigations are completed in coroner's cases, the coroner will provide documentation to the mortuary authorising the deceased's release. The coroner can open and adjourn an inquest if one is required, to allow the deceased to be released in a timely fashion. They will also contact the family to inform them of the post-mortem findings and instruct the assigned funeral director to collect the deceased or prompt the family to do so. Mortuary staff will ensure that outstanding tissues relating to the deceased are handled in accordance with the wishes of a person in a suitably qualified relationship with the deceased's (sometimes referred to as next of kin) prior to release of the body in all cases.

In non-coronial cases the hospital bereavement office team will assist in the generation of the correct release forms, burial orders and cremation forms. They will also inform the family and funeral director as required. Bereavement services will also take a lead role in cases where no next of kin is present. These cases are often referred to local authority services for cremation/funeral and require additional work to ensure that the deceased is handled efficiently and with respect.

Once informed, the assigned funeral director will liaise with mortuary staff to gain any further information they may require and inform them of a likely collection date. Some mortuaries will pre-emptively measure the height and width of the deceased to assist the funeral director in ordering and preparing a coffin. Most APTs will also assist the attending funeral director staff with any manual handling of the deceased onto their trolleys and moving equipment to ensure safety and respect.

Current Challenges

The sensitive nature of the work of mortuaries makes it a challenging and fulfilling role. Ensuring the correct staff numbers, skillset and staff retention is always a difficult balancing act for the management of these services. New staff may not find the role to be what they expected, and turnover is high. Media representation of mortuaries is rarely accurate, which does not help with the recruitment or retention of staff.

One of the current challenges for mortuary services is a national shortage of trained post-mortem pathologists. Without enough histopathologists, mortuaries may not have enough capacity to provide a timely service. Some histopathologists choose not to perform post-mortem examinations, for a variety of reasons. There has been some preliminary work done to investigate the introduction of advanced practitioner roles for APTs, as has been successfully introduced for other staff groups such as biomedical scientists, but this is at a very early stage.

In any event, mitigations will have to be put in place in the short to medium term, as the number of deaths varies throughout each year and the inability to process the work efficiently causes delays, which causes a backlog, which in turn causes storage problems, even for the larger mortuaries. In common with many mortuaries' plans for business continuity, the NNUH mortuary holds an additional 54 demountable temporary spaces for periods of peak activity, which does mitigate some storage issues, but the mortuary still has to utilise additional, logistically difficult, temporary storage either on or off site a number of times in the year.

During the COVID pandemic, tens of thousands of additional temporary spaces were put in place in mortuaries, aircraft hangars, temporary buildings and other locations around the country, and many remain in place.

Future Development of Mortuaries

The way that mortuaries function will likely have to change in line with the workload, demand, coroner's rules, HTA regulations and continuing lack of histopathologists. There are likely to be opportunities for mortuaries to combine with neighbouring facilities and even the possibility of the development of a regional service, as recommended in Peter Hutton's 2015 review of forensic pathology services in England and Wales.[8]

Some mortuaries already use post-mortem CT scans as an alternative or adjunct to invasive post-mortems, especially in areas where there is a high religious or cultural drive for them. In all likelihood more mortuaries will adopt CT scanning and digital pathology in the future. With the continuing fall in pathologist numbers in the UK the reporting of such cases may be digitally distributed to available pathologists or radiologists around the world. There are still some circumstances in which a conventional post-mortem is required – for instance, cases where the medical findings aren't conclusive on CT imaging.

Conclusions

The function of mortuaries is complex and sensitive. Anatomical pathology technologists have and continue to develop a wide range of valuable skills to enable them to support the bereaved.

REFERENCES

1. Fisher P. Houses for the Dead: The Provision of Mortuaries in London, 1843–1889, 2009. http://www.stgitehistory.org.uk/media/housesforthedead.pdf (accessed 20 December 2021).
2. Royal Society for Public Health. Training in Anatomical Pathology Technology, 2021. https://www.trainingapt.com/ (accessed 20 December 2021).
3. Human Tissue Authority. The Regulator of Human Tissue and Organs, 2021. https://www.hta.gov.uk/ (accessed 20 December 2021).
4. The National Archives. The Report of the Public Inquiry into Children's Heart Surgery at the Bristol Royal Infirmary 1984–1995, 2001. https://webarchive.nationalarchives.gov.uk/ukgwa/20100407202128/http://www.dh.gov.uk/en/Publicationsandstatistics/Publications/PublicationsPolicyAndGuidance/DH_4005620 (accessed 20 December 2021).
5. The House of Commons. The Royal Liverpool Children's Inquiry Report, 2001. https://assets.publishing.service.gov.uk/government/uploads/system/uploads/attachment_data/file/250934/0012_ii.pdf (accessed 20 December 2021).
6. Human Tissue Authority. The Human Tissue Act 2004, 2020. https://www.hta.gov.uk/guidance-professionals/hta-legislation/human-tissue-act-2004 (accessed 20 December 2021).
7. NHS England. Blood and Transplant, 2021. https://www.nhsbt.nhs.uk/ (accessed 20 December 2021).
8. GOV.uk. A review of forensic pathology in England and Wales, 2015. https://assets.publishing.service.gov.uk/government/uploads/system/uploads/attachment_data/file/477013/Hutton_Review_2015__2_.pdf (accessed 20 December 2021).
9. Human Tissue Authority. The Human Tissue Act 2004: A guide for the public. https://content.hta.gov.uk/sites/default/files/2020-12/Public%20guide%20to%20HTA%20Legislation.pdf?msclkid=3d451080af7e11eca85b004049d98950

CHAPTER 18

The Medical Reviewer System in Scotland

George Fernie

Introduction

In addition to having a separate legal jurisdiction and not possessing a coronial system, healthcare in Scotland is devolved to the Holyrood Parliament, so it was unsurprising that reform of death certification and review of Medical Certificates of Cause of Death (MCCDs) should take a different approach, whilst sharing a common aim with the other home nations in the UK.

The Brodrick Committee[1] reported in 1965, when its terms of reference were to review:

(i) the law and practice relating to the issue of Medical Certificates of the Cause of Death and for the disposal of dead bodies and;
(ii) the law and practice relating to coroners and coroners courts, the reporting of deaths to the coroners and related matters, and to recommend what changes are desirable.

The impetus for setting up this committee was provided by the publication of a report prepared by some of the British Medical Association's Forensic Medicine Sub-committee. The report, entitled 'Deaths in the Community', argued that such were the loopholes in the existing law regulating death certification and the coroners' system generally, that it was possible for homicides to go undetected, a claim the committee dismissed quite early into their investigations.

Subsequently, the Luce Review[2] identified some '*critical weaknesses of the death certification and coronial processes*' and although this report to which the author gave evidence on behalf of the BMA was not applicable to Scotland, many of the issues described were equally relevant.

Burial and Cremation Review Group

The Burial and Cremation Review Group,[3] under the chairmanship of Sheriff Robert Brodie, was established in 2005 with the outline remit '*to review the Cremation Acts of 1902 and 1952 (and the Cremation (Scotland) Regulations 1935, as amended, and the Burial Grounds (Scotland) Act 1855, as amended), and to make*

Table 18.1   The recommendations on death certification of the Burial and Cremation Review Group[3]

1. The procedure for certifying deaths should be sensitive to the many different faiths and beliefs in Scotland and ensure as short a delay as possible between death and disposal.
2. The same certification requirements should apply to all deaths regardless of the method of disposal of the body.
3. Any partner in a multi-GP practice who has access to information about the deceased may certify death. Any medically registered member of the Hospital team caring for and having information about the deceased may certify death.
4. Relatives should not have to pay for the forms required for the disposal of the body.
5. Appropriately trained professional groups such as registered nurses and paramedics should be entitled to verify the fact that life is extinct.
6. The office of medical referee at crematoria should be abolished.
7. A statistician to be called a Deaths Investigator should be appointed to enable frequent regular statistical checks to be carried out on all death data.
8. A new system of death certification should be introduced based on one or other of two models proposed by the Group.
9. One Model involves the appointment of Medical Investigators whose function will be to carry out a comprehensive paper-based scrutiny of a 1% random sample of all deaths and up to a further 1% of deaths where concerns have been expressed. In this model only one signature will be required to certify death apart from the deaths which have been subject to comprehensive scrutiny where the death certificate will require to be countersigned by the Medical Investigator.
10. The other Model involves the appointment of Medical Examiners whose function will be to carry out a basic scrutiny of all deaths and a comprehensive scrutiny of 1–2% of these deaths. The death certificate in all deaths will require to be countersigned by the Medical Examiner.

recommendations on how the legislation could be changed in order to better serve the needs of the people of Scotland. This work should, where appropriate, recognise the established role of the Procurator Fiscal Service, and take account of policy developments in England (specifically the Shipman Inquiry's work on death certification) and international good practice.'

The recommendations of the Review Group are shown in Table 18.1.

Presciently, there was a specific proposal in relation to pandemic flu/epidemic/infectious disease that was to allow for the power to suspend regulations relating to cremation in the case of a pandemic, epidemic or for any other reason and that this should be extended to apply to burials. This power should be sufficiently flexible to apply to the whole of Scotland or to a specified area.

Vale of Leven Inquiry

Whilst the stimulus for change in England and Wales was the failings identified within the Shipman Inquiry,[4] the final motivation in Scotland to bring in the necessary revision was the Vale of Leven Inquiry,[5] which published its report in 2014 having deliberated for five years. This highlighted the need for improved death certification amongst a number of other important improvements.

Primarily, this inquiry looked at the deaths of patients as a consequence of an outbreak of *Clostridium difficile (C.diff)*, where Scotland's largest health board was heavily criticised for allowing this to occur.

The probe, led by Lord MacLean, looked into care at Dunbartonshire's Vale of Leven Hospital (VOLH) between 2007 and 2008. Of the 143 patients with *C. diff*, it was a contributory factor in 34 deaths.

Lord MacLean said NHS Greater Glasgow and Clyde (GGC) had '*badly let down*' patients. The health board apologised unreservedly for a '*terrible failure*'. The judge referred to '*serious personal and systemic failures*' but also made various recommendations in regard to the reform of death certification.

The Scottish Government produced national guidance following the VOLH outbreak to ensure that deaths in which healthcare-associated infections (HAI) played a part were accurately certified by medical staff. The guidance was distributed to NHS boards in September 2009, with an updated version issued in October 2014. The updated guidance[6] asked NHS boards to:

- have systems in place to ensure the infection control manager is informed when HAI is recorded on a death certificate
- ensure consistent and reliable systems are in place to identify, as a minimum, *C. diff* and MRSA-associated deaths
- conduct rapid event investigation, as a minimum, for all deaths where *C. diff* or *Staphylococcus aureus* bacteraemia contributed to the death
- develop processes to ensure weekly and quarterly death data from National Records of Scotland for *C. diff* and MRSA (as a minimum) are reported to the infection control manager
- establish liaison with the Procurator Fiscal to ensure more coordinated action
- ensure all certifying doctors are appropriately trained in completing death certificates.

Explicitly, the Scottish Government indicated a wish to work with NHS Education for Scotland (NES) to ensure that certifying doctors are trained appropriately to complete death certificates and to provide relevant information for non-certifying staff and the public. They also expressed an intent to work collaboratively with Healthcare Improvement Scotland, National Records of Scotland and NHS Education for Scotland to develop a robust review system that randomly selects and reviews death certificates for accuracy and quality and provides feedback on the outcome to all relevant parties. The plan was for this information to be used for multiple purposes, including ongoing education and training for certifying doctors.

In any event, there was a general consensus throughout the UK that the archaic systems in place were not working satisfactorily, were unfit for purpose in the twenty-first century and required to be reformed to restore the desired functionality without impinging on the ability of those who had suffered a bereavement to arrange the desired disposal of their loved ones.

The Way Forward

The two alternative models set out above in the Brodie Report were originally put forward based on medical statistical advice, which suggested either would achieve the desired results of quality improvement and public reassurance. However, by 2013 it had been proposed that to deliver the second element successfully, a sample rate of 28% in conjunction with those cases investigated by the Procurator Fiscal would be preferable as that would result in approximately half of all the deaths occurring in Scotland being subjected to some form of scrutiny. Subsequently, being mindful of possible adverse impact on grieving relatives *should* there be delays in processing the reviews, it was decided that initially a 14% random selection would suffice in conjunction with the educational role outlined within the legislation. There was always an awareness that, should it be required, this could be ramped up. Likewise, whilst a reduction would be feasible, the reality of delivering a 24/7, 365-day-a-year service meant that a certain critical mass of personnel would be necessary for reasons of sustainability.

There was also a clear realisation of the need for independence from the territorial health boards to ensure impartiality of reviews but a degree of local accountability, with the outcome being that three sites were chosen to provide cover throughout Scotland with Aberdeen, Edinburgh and Glasgow initially selected. Given that about 40% of deaths occurred in general practice and the remainder in secondary care, be that hospital or hospice, it was decided there would be merit in having a blend of experienced doctors from both of these sectors to staff the service. There was a prerequisite from the Act that any Medical Reviewer (MR) appointed should have been a [registered] medical practitioner for the five years prior to appointment. In reality, to have the negotiating skills to effect change with senior members of the profession, that is the *minimum* acceptable period required.

Implementation in Scotland

The Death Certification Review Service (DCRS) was established in 2015 to fulfil the legislative requirements within the Certification of Death (Scotland) Act 2011.[7]

The aim of the DCRS continues to be to improve:

- the quality and accuracy of Medical Certificates of Cause of Death (MCCD)
- public health information about causes of death in Scotland, and
- clinical governance issues identified during the death certification review process.

To achieve this, we:

- review a specified proportion of randomly selected MCCDs before registration of the death can take place (*standard case*)
- where appropriate, approve requests allowing families to make funeral arrangements whilst the review is still being processed (*advance registration*)

- help families who believe the cause of death detailed on the MCCD is inaccurate by carrying out a review at their request (*interested person* review)
- work collaboratively with National Records of Scotland and registrars of births, deaths and marriages to review MCCDs that are not randomly selected for review but where the registrar has concerns the MCCD may not have been completed correctly (*registrar referral*)
- provide educational support to certifying doctors by reviewing the next 6–10 MCCDs they write (*'for cause' review*), and
- administer and authorise the burial and cremation of people who have died outside the UK and are returned to Scotland for funeral (*repatriation*).

The DCRS does not review:

- the quality of care provided to the deceased prior to their death, and
- suspicious deaths or deaths that should be reported to the Procurator Fiscal under the Inquiries into Fatal Accidents and Sudden Deaths etc. (Scotland) Act 2016.

This focus of the DCRS work has been clear from the start and this has almost certainly reduced the numbers of 'interested person' reviews received where pre-launch, the anticipation was that many more such applications would be received; but even with understandable concerns in diagnoses during the COVID-19 pandemic, DCRS typically undertakes single-figures of these each year.

Likewise, the success of the DCRS has resulted in a minimal number of 'for cause' reviews, albeit a statistical justification for identifying individual doctors for such a requirement has been developed, were the management board minded to go down that route.

Random selection via a computerised algorithm at National Records for Scotland was designed to ensure the planned coverage through the country over a two-year period.

Measurement of Quality in the MCCD

In section 8 of the underpinning legislation, there is helpful provision of a metric with which to ascertain whether or not there has been improvement in the content of the MCCDs completed by certifying doctors and also how this should be performed. This stipulates:

Review of medical certificates of cause of death
A medical reviewer must review any medical certificate of cause of death—
referred under section 24A of the 1965 Act[8] or in respect of which an application has been made under section 4(1) (other than one which has been rejected as vexatious under section 4(3)).
In conducting a review, the medical reviewer may—

examine the health records of the deceased person to whom the certificate relates, seek the views of the medical practitioner who attested the certificate, make enquiries of any other person who the medical reviewer considers may have information about the health of the deceased person (for example, a member of the deceased person's family, a carer or a nurse), make such other enquiries and examine such other things as the medical reviewer considers appropriate.

Following a review under subsection (1) the medical reviewer must come to a view on whether the certificate is in order.

For the purposes of this Act, a certificate is in order where a medical reviewer is satisfied, on the basis of the evidence available to the medical reviewer (MR), that—

the cause (or causes) of death mentioned represents a reasonable conclusion as to the likely cause (or causes) of death, and the other information contained in the certificate is correct.

The Review Process

Originally, it had been planned for a single type of review to be undertaken but the Health and Sport Committee of the Scottish Parliament decided that there should be a more basic Level 1 scrutiny whereby the MR should consider the content of the MCCD and discuss this with the certifying doctor and a more detailed Level 2 consideration looking at the content of relevant material to corroborate what was written therein.

A deliberate decision was taken that there should be no requirement to view paper records, short of concerns in respect to their integrity, because of the associated governance risks in them going astray. Due to the advent of greater IT functionality there was consequential blurring of the types of review with a hybrid version being developed during the 2020 COVID-19 pandemic. Even at its inception, the service confirmed the identity of the deceased patient with a Community Health Index (CHI) lookup and an Emergency Care Summary (ECS) review to show prescribed drugs, and also did a GMC registration check to ensure the doctor did, indeed, have a licence to practise. Subsequently, with the extension of availability of meaningful content in the electronic key information summary (eKIS), where this markedly improved at the advent of the COVID-19 pandemic due to the need for better anticipatory care planning, this became a tool of choice for the reviewers and often supplied the confirmatory data required, even fairly late in that patient's life. That said, there may be a significant event that takes place in the final week of life where specific confirmatory material is required, and a scanned investigation or case note entry is then requested by the service.

The other 'game-changer' with reviews was the introduction of the electronically completed MCCD (eMCCD) in primary care and for hospices, where at the time of writing, software has been developed for the hospital sector but had not been switched on. This removed registrar errors from the system although paradoxically the 'not in order' rate was worse than with handwritten certificates, suggesting an IT literacy issue.

Figure 18.1 is taken from the Death Certification Review Service Annual Report 2019–2020[9] and shows the number of cases and breakdown of case type and outcome.

Outcome of 'Not in Order' Review

MCCDs are deemed to be 'not in order' if the certifying doctor makes a clinical or an administrative error.

A total of 1228 randomised reviews were found to be 'not in order' in 2019/20, 75% of which were found to have a clinical closure category recorded. Figure 18.2 provides a breakdown of all clinical errors. The most common error recorded was 'cause of death too vague', at 53%.

DCRS carried out analysis of the 'cause of death too vague and incorrect' category and found that the most common errors occur when defining:

- neoplasms (cancer) 7.5% of all reviews
- diseases of the circulatory systems (affecting the heart) 4.7% of all reviews
- diseases of the respiratory system (breathing) 2.0% of all reviews
- mental and behavioural disorders (dementia) 1.3% of all reviews.

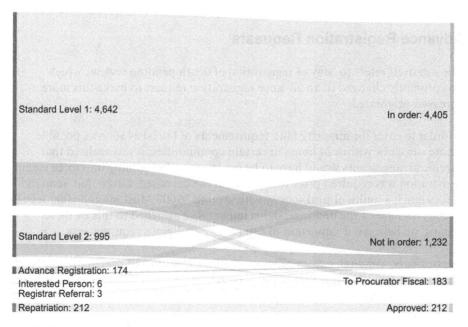

Figure 18.1   Sankey diagram of number of cases and breakdown of case type and outcome from the Death Certification Review Service Annual Report 2019–2020[9]

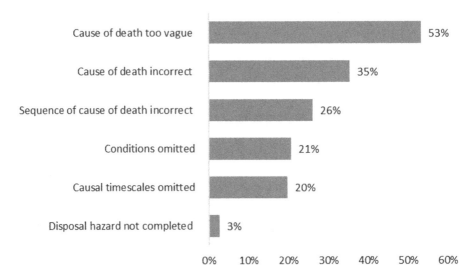

Figure 18.2   Bar chart of clinical categories recorded from the Death Certification Review Service Annual Report 2019–2020.[9]

If the MCCD is not accurate, the Medical Reviewer will request the certificate is amended or replaced by the certifying doctor. In 2019/20, 91.9% of reviews found to be 'not in order' required an email amendment whilst 8.1% of reviews required a replacement MCCD.

Advance Registration Requests

The Act itself refers to 'stay of registration of death pending review', which was promptly changed to an advance registration request to make this more bereaved-orientated.

In order to cater for minority faith requirements of burial as soon as possible, before sunset or within 24 hours in certain communities, it was realised that specific arrangements would have to be made as the Act coming into force meant registration was required prior to disposal of the deceased. Given that Scotland is very much a multicultural society with around 76 000 Muslims and 6000 Jewish people, because of the understandable importance attached to this by these groups, we believed it important to cater for any religious requirements.

Interestingly, although not for religious reasons, custom and practice in the North of Scotland and Islands is that burial should occur within 72 hours of a death and many applications have been on this basis.

If an MCCD is selected for review and the bereaved need the funeral to go ahead promptly, in special circumstances they may request advance registration. Special circumstances identified during the Scottish Government consultation included:

- if there are religious or cultural reasons to bury a person's body quickly
- if holding up the funeral would cause a lot of distress, and
- for other reasons, such as family have travelled from abroad for the funeral.

The service will usually approve or decline an advance registration application within two hours. If the application for advance registration is approved, the funeral can go ahead. If the application for advance registration is not approved, the funeral will have to wait until the Level 1 or Level 2 review is finished.

In essence, this means that burial can proceed but the specified type of review is still completed.

The main reason for declining an application is if it is obvious that a report to the procurator fiscal will be required, although significant deficiencies will also result in a request being rejected.

Proof of Concept

Whilst it was clear from the preparatory work that proportionate, random scrutiny should be able to improve the quality of MCCDs, it was not until DCRS effected reviews that we were able to confirm this strategy would be successful.

Figure 18.3 is a run chart from the DCRS annual report at the end of the fifth year of operation, which demonstrates that the system worked, without unnecessary delays that would impact on those who had lost a loved one and would not only allow the service to do this in a manner that was cost-effective but would

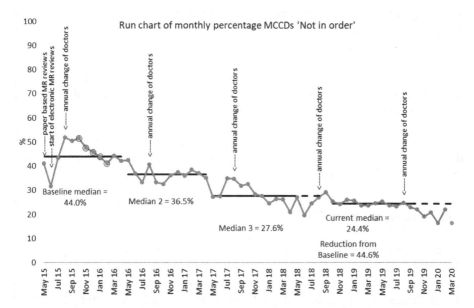

Figure 18.3   Run chart from the Death Certification Review Service Annual Report 2019–2020[9]

also do this nationally whilst at the same time producing better public health data and enhancing clinical governance.

Unanticipated Popularity

It had always been intended that DCRS would have an advisory function and in year 5, the service received 2644 enquiry calls. There are signs of further increase; in March 2020, the service received the maximum number of enquiry calls in one week at 294, and it is worth noting that 66 of these calls were COVID-19 related. This temporary increase was not sustained beyond the COVID-19 pandemic.

The number of self-motivated enquiry calls contrasted with mainly mandated reviews in that same period, at 6032, with advice requested being markedly more than anticipated at the inception of the service.

However, the view has been taken that the benefit accrued from this educational and supportive approach is one of the main reasons that certifying doctors have been so co-operative in their interactions with Medical Reviewers, meaning that formal escalation in terms of section 10 of the Act have been an absolute rarity.

Enlightened Decisions

Although the Act would permit a charge to be levied, the bold decision was that the delivery of the reviews would be free at the point of delivery in the same way as envisaged for other aspects of the NHS when it was first conceived. Doing so was in distinction to the Medical Examiner system in England and Wales, albeit they had an aspiration to review all the non-coronial MCCDs. When the new arrangements were implemented throughout the country, fees for cremation certificates were simultaneously abolished.

Another difference is that the service is independent of the territorial health boards whence the certificates are produced, ensuring impartiality and embracing clinical governance as a core function.

This does not mean one system is better or worse than the other, of course, but it is different, in the same way as the National Health Service has diverged across the home nations of the United Kingdom.

The Pandemic and Beyond

Under section 2(7) of the Certification of Death (Scotland) Act 2011, Scottish Ministers have the power to reduce the percentage of MCCDs randomised for review or suspend by order, the referral of certificates to the Medical Reviewer during an epidemic, pandemic or if it becomes necessary to do so to prevent the spread of infectious disease or contamination.

In response to the COVID-19 pandemic, the service worked closely with the Scottish Government, National Records of Scotland, Registrars and the Procurator Fiscal and changes from the 'normal' service were put in place to support:

- families and give public reassurance
- Health Boards and to reduce pressures on frontline staff
- Crown Office and Procurator Fiscal services to manage reports on deaths from COVID-19
- registrars to manage the significant increase in death registrations
- funeral directors to progress funerals quickly.

Timeline 2020

13 March Team start working from home to free up capacity within NHS24 sites to support NHS24 COVID-19 response team.

16 March Cessation of the requirement for repatriation paperwork to be certified.

22 March Percentage of randomised reviews was reduced to 4%.

23 March Suspension of the requirement to report deaths from COVID-19 to the Procurator Fiscal put in place.

27 March MCCD reviews suspended.

28 March Identified, through analysis of service enquiries, an understandable difference in the amalgamation of Health Protection Scotland (HPS) and NRS data. This supported the change in reporting by the Scottish Government on the actual number of COVID-19 related deaths being reported each day.

11 May MCCD reviews reinstated at 4% using a new hybrid Level 1 model which allowed the service to access the electronic key information summary (eKIS).

Although the pandemic extended into 2021, confidence in the ability to readily change the sample size allowed DCRS to keep functioning without a cessation of random reviews, meaning that although there was responsive variation throughout that year in the second wave, as normal a service as possible was maintained. By 10 May 2021, the types of review and percentage selection had returned to pre-pandemic specifications.

Conclusions

Scotland was the first of the home nations to reform medical certification of cause of death, which took place in 2015. This was done on time and under budget despite requiring a new IT system connecting two different governmental departments, National Records of Scotland and the NHS.

Notwithstanding the complexity, the new process has successfully improved the quality and accuracy of these important documents ensuring families have a much clearer understanding of why their loved ones died as well as providing improved public health data, which is something that assumed much greater significance with the unpredicted pandemic of 2020.

Importantly, all this has been done without imposing unnecessary delays on the ability to make funeral arrangements or impinge significantly on clinicians' ability to look after patients due to the educational approach that lies at the heart of the service.

REFERENCES

1. The National Archives. Committee on Death Certification and Coroners, 1965. https://discovery.nationalarchives.gov.uk/details/r/C9239 (accessed 20 December 2021).
2. Luce T. Fundamental Review of Death Certification and Investigation in England, Wales and Northern Ireland, 2001–03, 2006. https://publications.parliament.uk/pa/cm200506/cmselect/cmconst/902/902we02.htm (accessed 20 December 2021).
3. Burial & Cremation Review Group. Report and Recommendations, 2007. https://consult.gov.scot/burial-cremation/consultation-on-a-proposed-bill-relating-to-burial/supporting_documents/Burial%20and%20Cremation%20Review%20group.pdf (accessed 20 December 2021).
4. The National Archives. The Shipman Inquiry. 1st–6th Reports, 2002–2005. https://webarchive.nationalarchives.gov.uk/20090808155110/http://www.the-shipman-inquiry.org.uk/reports.asp (accessed 20 December 2021).
5. MacLean. The Vale of Leven Hospital Inquiry, 2014. https://hub.careinspectorate.com/media/1415/vale-of-leven-hospital-inquiry-report.pdf (accessed 20 December 2021).
6. GOV.scot. The Scottish Government's Response to the Vale of Leven Hospital Inquiry Report, 2014. https://www.gov.scot/publications/scottish-governments-response-vale-leven-hospital-inquiry-report/pages/7/ (accessed 20 December 2021).
7. GOV.uk. Certification of Death (Scotland) Act, 2011. https://www.legislation.gov.uk/asp/2011/11/contents (accessed 20 December 2021).
8. GOV.uk. Registration of Births, Deaths and Marriages (Scotland) Act, 1965. https://www.legislation.gov.uk/ukpga/1965/49/contents (accessed 20 December 2021).
9. Healthcare Improvement Scotland. Death Certification Review Service Annual Report, 2020. http://www.sad.uk.net/media/16518/20200519-dcrs-annual-report-2020.pdf (accessed 20 December 2021).

Further Reading

Cameron C, Gumbel E. *Clinical Negligence*. Oxford: Oxford University Press; 2007.

Coroners and Justice Act 2009 – downloadable from: www.legislation.gov.uk

Cremation Society. History of Cremation in the United Kingdom, 2019. https://www.cremation.org.uk/history-of-cremation-in-the-united-kingdom#:~:text=%201874%20-%201974%20%20 1%20Introduction.%20Probably,a%20paper%20entitled%20The%20Treatment%20of...%20 More%20 (accessed 20 December 2021).

Davies D, Mates L. *Encyclopaedia of Cremation*. London: Routledge; 2016.

Department of Health & Social Care. Integration and Innovation: Working together to improve health and social care for all, 2021. https://www.gov.uk/government/publications/working together-to-improve-health-and-social-care-for-all/integration-and-innovation workingtogether-to-improve-health-and-social-care-for-all-html-version (accessed 22 June 2021).

Dorries C. Coroners' Courts. *A Guide to Law and Practice (3rd edition)*. [2014]. Oxford University Press. ISBN 978-0-19-956611-2.

Duffy P. *Whistle in the Wind: Life, death, detriment and dismissal in the NHS. A whistleblower's story*, 1e. Independently published; 2019.

England J. *NHS Whistleblowing and the Law*. Law Brief Publishing; 2019.

Healthcare Improvement Scotland. Death Certification in Scotland, 2015. https://www.healthca reimprovementscotland.org/our_work/governance_and_assurance/death_certification.aspx (accessed 20 December 2021).

Healthcare Improvement Scotland. Death Certification in Scotland: COVID-19 useful information, 2020. https://www.healthcareimprovementscotland.org/our_work/governance_and_assur ance/death_certification/covid-19_useful_information.aspx (accessed 20 December 2021).

Hutton P, Mahajan R, Kellehear A. *Death, Religion and Law: A Guide For Clinicians*. New York: Routledge; 2019.

Lintern S. Chief Coroner warns over watered down medical examiner role, *Health Services Journal*, 20 December 2018. https://www.hsj.co.uk/policy-and-regulation/chief-coronerwarns-over-watered-down-medical-examiner-role/7024072.article (accessed 23 June 2021).

Luce T. Reform of the coroner system and death certification. Legislation is expected next month. *BMJ* 335 680–681 2007.

Matthews P. Jervis On Coroners. [2019]. Sweet and Maxwell (14th Edition). ISBN 97804 14072701.

McCorristine S (ed.). *Interdisciplinary Perspective on Mortality and Its Timings: When is Death?* London: Palgrave Macmillan; 2017.

NHS. Information for primary care on extending medical examiner scrutiny to non-coronial deaths in the community, online. https://www.england.nhs.uk/establishing-medical-examiner system-nhs/non-coronial-deaths-in-the-community/ (accessed 22 June 2021).

NHS England and NHS Improvement. System letter: Extending medical examiner scrutiny to non-acute settings, 2021. https://www.england.nhs.uk/wp-content/uploads/2021/06/B0477-extending-medical-examiner-scrutiny-to-non-acute-settings.pdf (accessed 22 June 2021).

National Medical Examiner for England and Wales. Implementing the Medical Examiner System: National Medical Examiner's good practice guidelines. January 2020. https://www.england.nhs.uk/wp-content/uploads/2020/08/National_Medical_Examiner_-_good_practice_guide lines.pdf (accessed 22 Jun 2021).

National Quality Board. National Guidance on Learning from Deaths, 2017. https://www.eng land.nhs.uk/wp-content/uploads/2017/03/nqb-national-guidance-learning-from-deaths.pdf (accessed 20 December 2021).

NHS Scotland. Support Around Death, 2021. https://www.sad.scot.nhs.uk (accessed 20 December 2021).

NME Good Practice Series publications https://www.rcpath.org/profession/medical-examiners/good-practice-series.html

Office for National Statistics. Guidance for Doctors Completing Medical Certificates of Cause of Death in England and Wales, 2020. https://assets.publishing.service.gov.uk/government/uploads/system/uploads/attachment_data/file/877302/guidance-for-doctors-completingmedical-certificates-of-cause-of-death-covid-19.pdf (accessed 22 June 2021).

Parsons B. *The Evolution of the British Funeral Industry in the 20th Century: From Undertaker to Funeral Director*. Bingley: Emerald; 2018.

Royal College of Pathologists. Cause of Death List, 2020. https://www.rcpath.org/uploads/assets/c16ae453-6c63-47ff-8c45fd2c56521ab9/G199-Cause-of-death-list.pdf (accessed 22 June 2021)

Royal College of Pathologists. National Medical Examiner's Good Practice Series No.3, 2021. https://www.rcpath.org/uploads/assets/daf86eaa-d591-40d5-99d54118d10444d2/Good-Practice-Series-Learning-disability-and-autism-For-Publication.pdf (accessed 20 December 2021).

Rugg J, Parsons B. *Funerary Practice in England and Wales*. Bingley: Emerald Publishing; 2018.

Samanta J. *Medical Law Concentrate*. Oxford: Oxford University Press; 2021.

Index

Note: Page references in *italic* refer to tables or figures.

Q

R

Printed in the United States
by Baker & Taylor Publisher Services